HEARTBEAT OF HOPE

A mother's journey through
resilience, medicine and hope

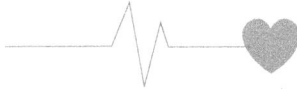

Ezinwanne Lilian Ozuloha

Conscious Dreams
P U B L I S H I N G

Heartbeat of Hope

First Printed in United Kingdom, 2025

Published by Conscious Dreams Publishing
www.consciousdreamspublishing.com

Edited by Elise Abram

Typeset by Oksana Kosovan

ISBN: 978-1-917584-27-2

Dedication

To my brave son, Lion:

For your incredible strength, unyielding resilience, and the light you bring into my life. You are the heartbeat of this story and the inspiration behind every word. This book is my tribute to you, a testament to your bravery, resilience and the hope you have given us all.

And to all the parents and families facing health challenges with their children or loved ones:

This book is for you, for every sacrifice, every sleepless night and every step forward in hope and love. May you find strength, healing and light on your journey.

Table of Contents

A Mother's Intuition

I never imagined that a routine 20-week ultrasound scan would change my life forever. Like any expectant mother, I walked into the hospital with my heart full of excitement and nerves, eager to see my baby's tiny form on the screen, but in an instant, joy turned to dread the moment the sonographer's expression shifted, and I knew something was terribly wrong.

Before she even spoke, a cold wave of fear washed over me. My baby's heart was not like other hearts; that is what the doctors would soon tell me. In that single moment, my world collapsed into chaos, a maelstrom of fear and uncertainty. I could not have imagined the strength I would need to repeatedly summon just to survive the days ahead. What I did not know yet was that the journey

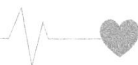

would push me to my limits, test every ounce of faith I had and redefine the very meaning of hope.

As a mother of two, I had already faced the highs and lows of parenthood, but nothing could have ever prepared me for this. I was about to step into a world of relentless medical tests, endless appointments and a crushing uncertainty that would push me to the brink of breaking.

This is my story, but it is more than that. It is a story for every parent who has ever been told their child must face a battle they never saw coming. This is for the mothers and fathers who stand helpless and terrified yet find the strength to hold it all together for the ones they love.

Nonetheless, this story is not just for parents. It is for anyone who is ever faced with the unthinkable: an illness, a loss or an unexpected challenge that turns your life upside down. We all have those moments when the ground beneath us crumbles, and we are forced to confront our deepest fears. In those moments, it is easy to feel isolated and as though no one else could understand, but in those dark hours, we discover our ability to be resilient and a strength we never knew we had. We are not alone in our struggles. Our stories may differ, but the threads of hope connect us all, weaving a tapestry of shared experience and unshakable faith.

This is not just a mother's story; it is a story of humanity, of what it means to stand at the edge of despair and fight your way back. It is a testament to the power of hope, community and the unwavering strength we find in the people who stand by our sides when the world falls apart.

Join me on this journey, not just through the pain but through the triumphs that come when we embrace resilience in the face of overwhelming odds. Together, we will discover that hope is not just a fleeting feeling. It is a force, a heartbeat that propels us through the darkest days, reminding us that even in the face of life's greatest storms, we can—and will—survive.

This is where my story begins, with a storm I never saw coming, a storm that changed everything. Yet, through it all, I learned about resilience, love, medicine, and, most importantly, the unshakable power of hope.

This is my journey, and it starts here.

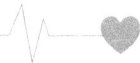

CHAPTER 1

Unexpected News

As I was already a mother of two, pregnancy was not new to me, but this time felt different from the start. I was a second-year social work student, juggling the regular responsibilities of life, including work placement, assignments and parenting. However, nothing could have prepared me for what unfolded at my 20-week ultrasound scan.

While I settled into the familiar rhythm of motherhood, balancing the daily needs of my two young children, Milo, four, and Hugo, two, I found myself back at the hospital for what was supposed to be a routine 20-week scan for my third baby. One of my best friends, Ava, came along with me, full of excitement. She was already planning a surprise baby shower and gender reveal. Loving

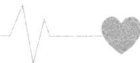

surprises as she did, she insisted on knowing the baby's gender ahead of time so she could plan every detail of the shower, right down to the colours and theme, with the perfect individualised touch.

It was a moment filled with light-heartedness, joy and that unique thrill of not knowing what was to come but still feeling so connected to it. I could not wait for the baby shower to reveal the gender, but for now, I was content with sharing the anticipation with Ava. We exchanged ideas as we sat in the waiting room, laughed and joked as if we were about to embark on a fun adventure rather than a medical appointment.

After a brief wait, a kind-looking female sonographer called us into the ultrasound room. The room was dimly lit, casting a calm ambience over what was usually a nervous experience for me. Ava and I shared a smile as I settled onto the table, and my stomach was coated in that familiar, cool gel. The sonographer introduced herself, and I quickly explained that I wanted the gender to be kept a secret from me. Instead, Ava would be the keeper of the exciting news until the big reveal.

'Of course.' The sonographer smiled. 'I'll tell Ava the gender in a moment. You can step out of the room if

you'd like.' Her tone was easy-going, and everything felt normal. Routine, even.

As the scan began, I felt a wave of emotions. That familiar mix of excitement and anxiety washed over me as I watched the screen, hoping to see those precious little limbs and that tiny heartbeat flickering away. Every ultrasound felt like a glimpse into a hidden world, a private moment shared with this little being I had yet to meet but already loved with my whole heart. My thoughts raced with possibilities: Would the baby be a boy or a girl? Would he or she look like Tee, me or Milo and Hugo?

The sonographer's voice broke through my thoughts. 'It looks like your baby is in a bit of a tricky position.' She paused, reassuring me with a smile. 'But don't worry, this is perfectly normal. Babies sometimes get too comfortable—or just get sleepy and don't feel like moving.' She looked at the screen again before turning back to me. 'I'll give you a chance to step out for a bit. Sometimes a little movement helps them shift into a better position for a clearer view.'

I nodded, grateful for her calm demeanour. 'Sounds good.'

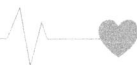

'Oh,' she added, glancing at Ava, who was standing quietly by the screen. 'This will also give me a chance to tell Ava the baby's gender. I think I've already spotted it.'

Ava and the sonographer exchanged a quick glance, their expressions lighting up with a shared secret. They whispered something to each other, their voices low and full of excitement. I smiled at their playful exchange, trying not to let my curiosity overtake me. It all felt so casual, so light-hearted—just another step along the way.

Moments later, as planned, I rose from the scan table, reaching for a tissue to gently wipe away the cool gel that lingered on my belly. With practiced ease, I smoothed down my T-shirt, letting the soft fabric fall back into place, covering the bare skin that had moments before cradled the sonographer's probe.

I stepped out to let Ava receive the big secret. I could see her face light up when I returned, her grin wide and eyes twinkling with mischief. She was so pleased with herself, holding on to the revelation like a precious gem she could not wait to show off. For me, though, it was still a game of patience, and I did not think much about anything beyond the joy of that day, the magic of seeing my baby and the quiet anticipation of what lay ahead.

I laid back down on the table and pulled up my t-shirt, exposing my belly once more. The sonographer reapplied the cool gel, spreading it evenly before pressing the probe gently against my skin. The sonographer resumed the scan, and her demeanour changed. She became quieter, more focused. Her brow slightly creased as she moved the probe across my belly, her eyes narrowing at the screen.

'I just need to take a few more measurements,' she said, her voice calm but noticeably more serious. 'Your baby's a little small, and I can't quite get a good look at everything today.'

Her words were nonchalant, but something shifted in the room. My heart skipped a beat as a seed of doubt planted itself in my mind. What wasn't she seeing? The carefree energy that had filled the room minutes ago faded. The sonographer suggested I rebook the appointment for two weeks, when the baby would be bigger and hopefully, in a better position for a clearer scan.

As Ava and I left the hospital, we were still excited about the baby shower and the gender reveal, but a quiet unease had settled over me that I could not shake, though I tried to push it aside and convince myself it was all routine. After all, these things happened all the time, right?

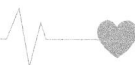

The weeks passed, and before I knew it, it was time for the follow-up ultrasound scan. That time, I went alone.

The sterile smell of the hospital hung in the air as I lay on the examination table, the cool gel spreading across my belly, momentarily jolting me from my thoughts. This was supposed to be a routine checkup, a joyous moment in my pregnancy. I couldn't help but feel a wave of excitement wash over me as I glanced at the monitor, eagerly expecting the image of the tiny life that had become the focal point of my existence.

I thought back to the moment I first learned I was pregnant. The sheer joy I felt, the dreams I began to weave around this new life, the hopes of baby showers, nursery colours, and even the sweet sound of coos that would soon fill our home again. That pregnancy felt like a beautiful journey despite the chaos of juggling two other children, Milo and Hugo, and my studies, but now, as the sonographer's brow furrowed, I sensed that something was not right.

'Everything okay?' I asked, my heart beginning to race. I was desperate to maintain a calm facade, but the unease gnawed at my insides.

The sonographer looked up, her expression shifting from concentration to concern. 'Let's just take a closer look at

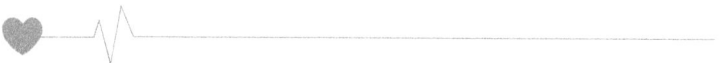

a few things,' she said, her tone professional yet laced with an undertone of urgency that sent my anxiety spiralling.

I swallowed hard, my palms clammy against the examination table. 'What do you mean?' I enquired, the tremor in my voice betraying my calm demeanour.

'Just a routine check,' she replied, though I could see the worry etched in her features. After several minutes, she said she was going to call in a senior colleague for a second opinion. My pulse quickened. I nodded, trying to keep calm, but I knew it was not just routine anymore. She left the room, and I was left alone, the silence stretching like an uncomfortable shroud around me. I forced myself to breathe, tried to push away the gnawing fear that had begun to settle in my chest.

Time seemed to stretch indefinitely as I lay there. I closed my eyes for a moment, focusing on the soft sounds of the hospital, the hum of machines, the rustle of paper, the faint murmur of distant voices, but instead of feeling comforted, I was haunted by the uncertainty of the moment.

What could be wrong? I could not shake the thought.

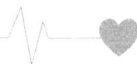

I reminded myself that this was just a precaution, that the sonographer might simply have wanted to ensure everything was fine.

Moments later, the sonographer returned, accompanied by a senior colleague. This new face was more experienced. She greeted me warmly, but her eyes were already on the screen. Her demeanour was calm but with an air of intensity that made my heart race even faster. 'We just want to double-check a few things,' she said, and I nodded, my stomach churning as they started examining the images on the screen again. They watched in silence, their faces serious yet professional, and I watched them, trying to read every glimmer of expression, every subtle glance they exchanged.

The atmosphere was thick with tension, and each click of the machine sounded like a countdown. I felt as if I were sitting in a storm, swirling with emotions: anxiety, confusion, fear. As they both scrutinised the screen, I could not help but feel as if I were being pulled deeper into the unknown, away from the bright expectations I once held.

After what felt like an eternity, the senior sonographer turned to me, her expression serious. 'There is something we are trying to look for in your baby's heart,' she began, choosing her words carefully. 'We cannot quite find it yet, but it could be nothing. We are going to refer you to a foetal cardiac medicine clinic for a more thorough examination.'

Her words hit me like a cold wave, sending a shiver through my body. A foetal cardiac medicine clinic? What did that mean? I sat there, the excitement of the past few weeks fading fast, replaced by a growing knot of worry. All I could think about was my baby. Was something wrong?

A rush of emotions flooded through me: panic, dread and a sense of impending doom. 'What does that mean?' I managed to ask, my voice a mere whisper.

'Don't panic,' she reassured me. 'It could be nothing, but we want to ensure that everything is thoroughly examined.' Her tone did little to soothe my fears; instead, it amplified them, feeding the anxiety that now felt all-consuming.

The once vibrant atmosphere from my earlier scan had vanished, replaced by a weighty silence. My mind raced. I felt as if the ground beneath me had shifted, and suddenly, I was standing on unfamiliar, unstable terrain. My hands trembled as I thanked the sonographer, and as she handed me the referral paperwork, I felt the weight of the world settle on my shoulders. 'They will schedule

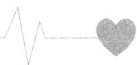

a detailed scan of your baby's heart, and they'll take a closer look,' she said, and I nodded numbly, though her words barely registered.

The reality of the situation crashed over me like a tidal wave. This was not how it was supposed to be. I had imagined the appointment as a simple checkup, a moment of joy, not the beginning of a journey into a realm of uncertainty and fear.

Once I stepped out of the hospital, the bright lights of the parking lot felt blinding. My legs felt heavy as I walked to my car, the burden of the news weighing me down. Alone in the quiet of the parking lot, tears spilt down my cheeks; each drop a mixture of fear and disbelief.

I fumbled for my phone, my hands trembling as I called Tee, my partner of well over a decade. His warm voice on the other end was a lifeline in my turbulent sea of emotions. 'Hey, babe,' he answered, his tone instantly concerned, 'what's wrong?'

I took a shaky breath, searching for the right words. 'The sonographer found something unusual in our baby's heart,' I managed to say, my voice quivering. 'They've referred me to a specialist.' The knot in my stomach tightened as I fought back tears.

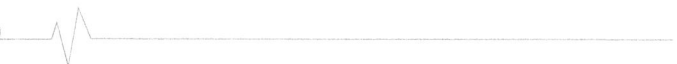

Tee's voice came through, steady and calm. 'All right, let us not jump to conclusions. It's probably nothing. Try not to worry too much.'

'I just… I don't know,' I said, my emotions spilling over. 'I'm scared.'

'Hey, don't be scared, babe,' he reassured me gently. 'Remember, no news is good news.'

I couldn't hold back the tears any longer. Through my sobs, Tee's concern was immediate and grounding. 'Can you drive home?' he asked, 'or do you want me to come pick you up? I could call a taxi for you.'

I took a deep breath, trying to gather myself. 'I think I can drive,' I replied, my voice a bit steadier, 'but I really wish you were here right now.'

'I wish I could be, too,' he said softly. 'Just take your time. Drive safely, okay? We'll talk more when you get home.'

'Okay,' I said, feeling a small sense of reassurance start to wash over me. 'I love you.'

'I love you more,' he replied, his voice filled with warmth. 'You've got this.'

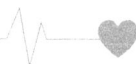

As I hung up, I took a deep breath, steeling myself for the drive ahead. The world outside felt muted, the vibrant colours dulled by the weight of my worry. I reminded myself that I needed to stay strong for my baby.

I started the car. The engine rumbled to life beneath me, but as I pulled out of the parking lot, my mind raced with thoughts. What could the 'unusual' finding in my baby's heart mean? I couldn't help but imagine the worst. What if my baby was sick? What if this was the beginning of a long, difficult journey? My heart raced as I gripped the steering wheel and tried to focus on the road ahead.

The drive home felt agonisingly long. Each stoplight stretched out; each moment dragged like a weight tied to my chest. I watched the world pass by, people going about their lives, blissfully unaware of the storm brewing inside me. I caught glimpses of mothers with their little ones, couples holding hands, laughter echoing from nearby parks. Each sight brought a pang of longing mixed with fear—what if my family never looked like that?

Tears blurred my vision as I fought to keep it together. I had to remind myself that I was not alone in this. I had Tee and my other children, and we would face whatever came together. I replayed his words in my mind—'It's probably nothing'—but how could I accept that? My

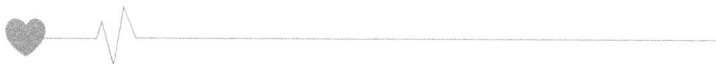

heart whispered doubts that echoed louder than the reassurances. What if it was something serious? What if I were walking into a nightmare? The what-ifs raced through my head like a relentless tide, each wave crashing against my fragile sense of peace.

Finally, I arrived home, but the familiar surroundings offered little comfort. When I arrived home, Tee had already picked up our two children, Milo and Hugo, from school and nursery. As I stepped inside, I was greeted by the chaos of everyday life, the sounds of my children playing, the remnants of their snacks scattered across the kitchen counter. For a moment, I felt a pang of guilt. They were so young, so innocent, and I could not help but feel as if I were about to shatter their world.

I took a deep breath, trying to centre myself. I knew I needed to stay strong for them. I was not just a mother to one; I was a mother to three. I could not let this consume me; I needed to be present for my children.

The kids came running towards me, their faces lighting up as they saw me. 'Mummy!' they shouted in unison, wrapping their arms around my waist. Their laughter filled the air, but it felt distant, muffled by the weight of my worry. I hugged them tightly, allowing their warmth

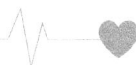

to seep into my bones, offering me a temporary reprieve from the chaos in my mind.

'Hi, loves,' I said, forcing a smile as I knelt to their level. 'Did you have fun?'

'Yeah! We played dinosaurs,' my youngest, Hugo, exclaimed, his eyes wide with excitement.

'*Roar*!' I said, mimicking a dinosaur. Their laughter erupted, momentarily lifting the heaviness in my heart, but the fleeting joy was bittersweet, a reminder of what was at stake.

'How was the appointment, Mum?' Milo asked eagerly. 'Did you see the baby? Is it a boy or a girl?'

I managed a smile as I pulled out the ultrasound photo. 'Here's your little brother or sister,' I said, handing it to them. They both stared at the image, full of curiosity and wonder.

'When will we know if it's a boy or a girl?' Hugo chimed in.

'In about a month, at the baby shower. Auntie Ava is planning a big surprise for us.'

They seemed satisfied with that, their excitement distracting them from my quiet worry.

I excused myself to the kitchen, where I could gather my thoughts without the children noticing my distress. As I poured myself a glass of water, I caught a glimpse of my reflection in the window. The worry etched across my face was a stark contrast to the vibrant life surrounding me. I took a moment to compose myself, forcing a smile.

Tee entered the kitchen shortly after, his face lighting up as he entered. 'Hey, babe,' he called, sweeping me into his arms. I relished the warmth of his embrace, the way it grounded me in the present, but as he pulled away and looked into my eyes, I saw concern flicker in his gaze.

'Let's talk,' he said gently, leading me to the living room couch. I took a deep breath, my heart racing as I prepared to share the weight of my fears with him. This was it, the moment I'd dreaded and anticipated all at once. The uncertainty I'd been carrying since leaving the hospital came rushing back, and I felt tears threatening to spill once more.

As we sat down on the couch, I took a moment to gather my thoughts. I glanced at our children playing nearby, blissfully unaware of the storm brewing in my heart. 'The

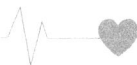

sonographer found something unusual in our baby's heart,' I started, my voice trembling slightly. 'She referred me to a specialist for a detailed scan.'

Tee's expression shifted from concern to focus. 'What kind of unusual? Did she say what it might be?' His brow furrowed as he leaned in closer, his hands clasped tightly together.

'She didn't go into specifics,' I said, my voice breaking. 'just that they saw something they wanted to take a closer look at. I don't know what that means, but...' I paused, the words catching in my throat, 'I'm scared, Tee.'

He reached for my hand and squeezed it reassuringly. 'I'm here, okay? We'll get through this together. You're not alone.'

The sincerity in his voice helped anchor me, but I couldn't shake the growing dread gnawing at my insides. 'What if it's something serious?' I whispered, my voice barely audible. 'What if our baby is sick?'

'Let's not jump to conclusions,' Tee replied, his tone steady but gentle. 'It could be nothing. You know how these things can be. Sometimes, they just want to be extra cautious.'

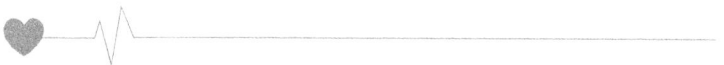

I nodded, knowing he was trying to reassure me, but the uncertainty lingered like a dark cloud. 'I just didn't expect this,' I admitted. 'I thought everything was fine. I thought I'd leave today with good news, not this.'

'I know,' he said softly. 'but you're strong. You've been through so much already. You'll handle this just like you've handled everything else. We're a team.'

As he spoke, I tried to let his words sink in, but my mind kept racing. I remembered the look on the sonographer's face, the way she'd hesitated before handing me the referral. I wondered if she saw something significant, something that would change everything.

'What if it's a heart problem?' I blurted, the thought suddenly taking shape in my mind. 'What if the baby has a serious condition?'

Tee's expression tightened. 'We'll cross that bridge if we come to it. Right now, let's focus on the next steps. When's the appointment?'

'Next week,' I said, the weight of the impending visit heavy in my chest. 'It feels so far away, yet so close. I wish I could just fast forward to that day and know what's going on.'

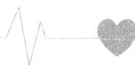

'Maybe we can distract ourselves until then,' Tee suggested. 'Let's do something fun as a family this weekend. We could go to the park or have a movie night.'

The idea of spending quality time with our children brought a flicker of warmth to my heart, and I nodded slowly. 'That sounds nice. I want to be present for them, but it's hard to push this out of my mind.'

'I get that,' he replied, his eyes softening. 'Just take it one day at a time. We can handle whatever comes our way together. We've built this life and family, and we'll navigate whatever challenges arise.'

As we sat there hand in hand, I felt a mix of gratitude and fear—gratitude for having Tee by my side and fear for what lay ahead. I knew this wasn't just about me anymore; it was about our family, our future and the precious life growing inside me.

That night, following the usual bedtime routine, as Milo and Hugo were in bed asleep, I found myself sitting in the living room replaying the day over and over in my mind. Sitting on the couch, I grabbed my phone and started searching online, looking up anything I could find about referrals to foetal cardiac specialists. Each article, each forum post, seemed to deepen my anxiety. There were so many possibilities, so many unknowns.

I lost track of time, reading until Tee interrupted me. 'You should get some rest,' he said gently. 'You have placement in the morning, and you need to be sharp for it. Don't let this stress you out, okay? We'll get through whatever happens.'

I nodded, though I wasn't sure I believed my own response. How could I rest when there was so much uncertainty? Still, I knew he was right. I had to keep going for my children, for myself, for our baby.

I lay in bed that night, but sleep didn't come easily. My mind was consumed with questions: What would the specialist say? What if something were seriously wrong with my baby's heart? What if...

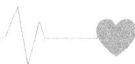

CHAPTER 2

The Diagnosis

The next week felt as if it stretched endlessly on, each day dragging as though time itself had slowed. I tried to stay occupied, focusing on the needs of my children, immersing myself in their laughter and play, but no matter how hard I tried, the looming uncertainty cast a dark shadow over even the brightest moments. I watched them as they created new memories, their carefree joy a stark contrast to the heavy burden of worry I carried within me. Guilt gnawed at me for not being fully present and for the silent fears I harboured that I couldn't share.

Finally, the day of the foetal cardiac medicine appointment arrived. Tee had taken the day off work to be with me, his steadfast support a lifeline in my storm of emotions. As we got ready to leave, dread began to settle deep in my

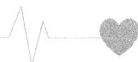

chest. I dressed carefully, choosing a soft grey two-piece outfit, hoping that something as simple as comfortable clothes could offer me a silver of calm. We dropped off Milo and Hugo at school and nursery before heading to the clinic. It was a morning appointment, and we hoped to return in time to pick up the boys.

The drive to the clinic was enveloped in a thick, tense silence. I found myself gripping the seatbelt tightly as if that could somehow contain the anxiety building inside me. Tee reached over and placed his hand gently on my knee, his touch grounding me. 'We're almost there,' he said softly. 'Just remember to breathe.'

I nodded and inhaled deeply in an attempt to centre myself as we pulled into the clinic's parking lot. The building stood ahead, sterile and intimidating, a stark reminder of how significant the day could be. As we walked inside, I couldn't shake the overwhelming sense that our lives were about to change in ways I couldn't yet imagine.

The waiting room was filled with other expectant parents, their faces showing a mixture of hope, excitement, and anxiety. I tried to focus on the faint sound of children laughing from a nearby play area, but my thoughts were consumed by fear—what if the news was bad? What if everything changed for us that day?

After what felt like an eternity, we were finally called into the examination room. The foetal sonographer greeted us with a warm smile, but there was a seriousness in her eyes that made my heart race. 'Thank you for coming in today,' she said, kindly but firmly. 'Let's take a look at your baby's heart and see what we can find.'

I lay down on the examination table, my pulse quickening as the sonographer began the scan. The rhythmic sound of the ultrasound machine filled the room, but the moments stretched into a painful silence. I watched her carefully examine the images, her brow furrowing with concentration, and I felt the weight of her unspoken words.

Finally, she turned to us, her expression both serious and compassionate. 'I've completed the scan,' she said gently. 'There's something unusual with your son's heart.'

Tee and I exchanged a glance as her words slowly sunk in.

Our son.

A boy.

We hadn't known the gender of our baby before then, and the realisation hit me hard. My heart sank, and tears welled up in my eyes, but I couldn't find the words to

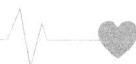

respond. The sonographer noticed our reactions and quickly apologised. 'I'm so sorry,' she said. 'I should have asked if you knew the gender.'

I managed a small nod. 'We were planning a surprise gender reveal next month,' I replied, my voice barely above a whisper. I looked at Tee and said softly, 'We're having another boy.'

Tee's face, usually so calm, looked pale and worried. He squeezed my hand gently. His voice was steady despite the fear in his eyes. 'Yes, another boy,' he said quietly.

I held his hand tighter, trying to reassure him—and myself—saying, 'We'll get through this, even though it feels like we're drowning.'

The sonographer told us to head to the waiting area while we waited for the doctor to review the scan. Tee helped me off the table. My legs felt heavy, as if they might give out beneath me. My mind raced as I realised we wouldn't make it in time to pick up the boys from school and nursery. 'Tee, we need to call someone to pick up the boys,' I said, my voice shaky.

I reached for my phone and tried to call Willow, our family friend, but there was no answer. Tee called Ethan,

Willow's husband, and when Ethan picked up, Tee handed me the phone.

'Hello, Ethan,' I said, trying to hold back my tears. 'We're running late... could you pick up the boys up from school and nursery?' but before I could finish, the words caught in my throat, and tears spilt down my face.

Ethan must have sensed my distress because he reassured us calmly, 'Don't worry. We've got it covered. We'll pick them up and take them home until you're ready.'

Tee took the phone, thanking Ethan before hanging up. We walked back to the waiting area holding hands; both of us lost in our thoughts. The silence between us was thick, heavy with the weight of unspoken fears.

As we sat down to wait for the doctor, I turned to Tee, my voice barely audible, and I said, 'What do you think the problem is?'

He looked at me, his expression unreadable. 'I don't know, babe,' he said quietly. 'Let's wait for the doctor. Try not to stress until we know more.'

We sat there in silence, but it felt like an eternity. The weight of the unknown pressed down on us. All we could

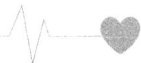

do was wait for the next piece of news that was likely to change our lives.

After what felt like an endless wait, we were finally called into the cardiac consultant's office. As we walked in, it felt as though my legs would barely support me. Inside the room were seven individuals, who each introduced themselves: the cardiac consultant, the cardiologist on call, her assistant, the paediatrician on call, a nurse, the midwife, and a nursing assistant. Seeing so many health professionals gathered in one room made my heart sink. I couldn't help but wonder why there were so many of them. Was it that serious?

'Hello, Mum and Dad,' the cardiac consultant greeted us, her kind eyes radiating both warmth and quiet confidence. She introduced herself and began reviewing the scan and pregnancy notes. 'We want to discuss what we've found,' she said gently, her voice steady but filled with gravity.

I saw concern spread across her face, and my heart pounded in my chest. My breath hitched as she began to explain the findings from the scans.

'Thank you for coming in today,' she said, her tone calm but firm. 'I want to go over what we've found and discuss the next steps.'

I nodded, feeling a lump form in my throat, barely able to ask, 'What exactly did you find?' My voice was shaky, betraying the torrent of emotions surging within me.

The cardiac consultant took a deep breath and looked at us with a steady gaze. 'We have some concerns about your baby's heart,' she said. 'The scans show a complex congenital heart defect called pulmonary atresia with a ventricular septal defect (VSD) and major aortopulmonary collaterals (MAPCAs). Your baby's heart is different from a typical heart.'

Her words hit me like a tsunami. I struggled to grasp the medical terms swirling around in my mind: pulmonary atresia, VSD, MAPCAs. In utter shock, I barely managed to ask, 'What is that, and what does it mean for my baby?'

'The pulmonary artery, which carries blood from the heart to the lungs, has not fully developed in your baby's heart. This is what we refer to as pulmonary atresia,' she explained slowly as if giving me time to absorb each word. 'Additionally, there is a hole between the two ventricles of the heart called a ventricular septal defect or VSD, which makes the situation more complex. The presence of MAPCAs means that your baby's body is trying to compensate by creating alternative vessels to get

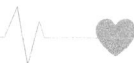

oxygenated blood to the lungs, but these vessels are not a long-term solution.'

I blinked, trying to wrap my head around what she was saying. My mind raced with more questions than I knew how to voice. 'Will my baby need surgery?' I finally asked, my voice filled with both fear and hope.

The doctor's voice was calm but filled with gravity steady but firm and now soft yet firm as she delivered the news. 'Yes,' she said, meeting our eyes with a calm steadiness. 'Most likely, the surgery will need to happen soon after birth. The structural issues in your baby's heart require early intervention. It's crucial to improving the outcome.'

She outlined the procedure and its risks, and it felt as if the ground was crumbling beneath me. A whirlwind of emotions—fear, sadness, and overwhelming uncertainty—hit me all at once. I glanced at Tee, whose face seemed to mirror my own feelings of worry and helplessness.

I swallowed hard, struggling to find my voice. 'Are there any other options?' I asked, almost in a whisper. 'What happens if we don't go through with the surgery?'

The cardiologist paused, her expression turning serious. 'Without surgery, the prognosis is poor. The heart won't be able to function properly, and sadly, your baby will not survive.'

Her words hit me like a punch to the chest. Desperate for any shred of hope, I felt my throat tighten as I asked, 'Is there any chance that everything might be, okay?'

She leaned in, her gaze steady and filled with quiet determination. 'There are many factors that affect the outcomes. While this is a serious condition, with surgery, many children can go on to lead healthy, fulfilling lives. Early intervention is our best chance to improve your baby's quality of life.'

She continued explaining the potential outcomes, and I felt despair creeping in and suffocating me. The future I had envisioned for my child seemed to be slipping away before it had even begun. What if he never had the chance to experience it?

Then, the conversation took an unexpected turn. The doctor's tone softened as she brought up something I wasn't prepared to hear: 'I know this is a lot to process,' she began gently. 'Given the complexity of your baby's condition, some families in similar situations consider

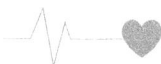

termination, especially because of the significant impact these challenges can have on the entire family.' She glanced at us, acknowledging the two other children we had. 'The extended hospital stays, surgeries, and the intensive care your baby would need might be very difficult on your family as a whole.'

I felt a wave of nausea wash over me, and my mind reeled, trying to process her words. I hadn't even considered termination. It felt like a gut punch, a suggestion that seemed out of place while explaining my baby's heart defects—why was she even bringing it up now?

The doctor continued, her voice steady but compassionate. 'Under the National Health Service guidelines, we cannot offer a termination after 25 weeks, even in cases of severe health challenges. Since you're currently at 24 weeks, I want to ensure you are fully informed of all your options so that you can decide soon, if needed.'

Hearing that, I felt like time was speeding up and everything was closing in. I was caught in a whirlwind of fear and disbelief, grappling with the weight of a decision I never imagined I'd have to face.

Tears welled in my eyes and streamed down my face as I shook my head vigorously. 'No,' I whispered, my voice cracking, 'I can't even think about that. This is my baby. I love him already, and I'm going to fight for him.'

The doctor nodded, her expression kind and understanding. 'I completely understand your concerns. We're here to support you, no matter what you decide. I want you to be fully aware of the challenges ahead, and while this journey will be difficult, know that we are committed to helping you in every way we can.'

Her words settled heavily on my heart. There was no escaping the reality we faced. This baby, our baby, needed us to be strong and fight for him, no matter how long or arduous the road ahead may be.

The doctor then added something that made my stomach churn: 'Given the complexity of your baby's heart condition, it's often accompanied by other congenital anomalies such as Trisomy 13, Down syndrome, and other abnormalities. It's important that we conduct further tests to check for any additional issues.'

I felt my breath catch as the seriousness of her words sank in. 'What does that mean?' I asked, my voice trembling.

'There could be other issues related to the heart condition,' she explained, her voice was calm but edged

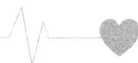

with hesitation. 'We need to do more testing to fully understand your baby's situation.'

The room seemed to close in on me as the weight of it all threatened to crush me. Tee's hand tightened around mine, his face a mask of worry. 'What do we do next?' he asked, his voice steady but tinged with fear.

'With your consent,' the doctor continued, 'we'll schedule an amniocentesis to check for genetic abnormalities, along with an echocardiogram to get a detailed view of your baby's heart. Amniocentesis is a procedure where we take a small sample of amniotic fluid from the womb, which contains your baby's genetic material. This test allows us to look for any chromosomal abnormalities or genetic conditions. While there is a small risk of miscarriage, it will provide us with a clearer understanding of your baby's overall health.'

I nodded, absorbing the significance of those words. The procedure sounded daunting, and the mention of the risks added to my fear.

The doctor continued, 'An echocardiogram is an ultrasound of your baby's heart. It will allow us to get a more detailed view of the heart's structure and function, so we can better understand the severity of the defects and plan the best course of action for surgery.'

I nodded numbly, feeling as if I were floating in a surreal bubble. The doctor's words washed over me, but all I could focus on was the uncertainty ahead. Each word felt like a drop of cold water splashing against my skin, awakening us to the stark reality of our situation. The doctor spoke in a tranquil tone as she explained the next steps, while my mind raced with questions and fears.

'I will book you in for the amniocentesis test,' the doctor continued, her tone matter-of-fact as she scribbled on a notepad. 'You should receive a letter in the post when the appointment has been scheduled.'

The appointment came to an end, disbelief hanging heavily in the air, making it hard to breathe.

Tee and I stood up and exited the clinic in silence. Each step towards the car felt like a march through a fog, my mind a whirlwind of emotions. The weight of the diagnosis pressed down on me, but beneath the fear, a fierce determination began to rise. I wouldn't let this dictate our journey; we would face it head-on together.

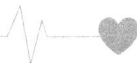

Once inside the car, I glanced at Tee, who sat in silence, lost in thought. 'What are you thinking?' I asked, my voice shaky.

'I'm just trying to wrap my head around everything,' he replied, his brow scrunched. 'This is a lot to take in, but we'll figure it out.'

I nodded, though uncertainty loomed over us like a storm cloud. 'I just can't believe this is happening. I thought everything would be fine. I thought we'd be celebrating, not...' My voice trailed off, tears spilling down my cheeks.

Tee reached over, taking my hand in his. 'We will get through this one step at a time. Let's take it day by day.'

Chapter 3

Telling Loved Ones

The journey back felt interminable. The minutes stretched into what felt like hours as we sat stuck in traffic. The diagnosis echoed in my mind like a relentless drumbeat, each thud pushing me deeper into a state of shock. Outside, the world moved on. Cars passed by pedestrians crossing the street, and the normal hum of life continued without pause. It felt like I was trapped in a separate world, one where nothing made sense anymore.

I took a deep breath and pulled out my phone, my hands trembling as I dialled Clara's number. She's my other best friend, the one who's always been a pillar of strength, and at the time, I needed that more than anything.

I took a shaky breath and whispered, 'Clara, it's me.'

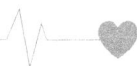

The concern in her voice was instant. 'Oh, no—what's wrong?'

I tried to hold it together, but the floodgates opened, and the tears flowed freely. 'I just got out of a doctor's appointment,' I said, my voice breaking. 'They diagnosed my baby with pulmonary atresia, VSD and MAPCAs.' Each word felt as if it was pulling me deeper underwater. 'The doctor said he'll need surgery as soon as he's born.'

Clara gasped softly. The silence that followed felt as if it would stretch on forever. 'I'm so sorry,' she said, her voice thick with emotion, mirroring the pain I felt. 'You and Tee don't deserve this. This isn't fair.'

In hearing her words, I felt an overwhelming sense of solidarity after hearing her words. Clara understood. She got it. She felt my pain. In that shared space of grief, I didn't feel quite so alone, but as we continued to talk, I noticed something shifting in Clara's tone. Despite the initial heartbreak, she began to find her footing, to pull herself together.

'Listen,' she said, her tone calm but resolute, 'You're strong, and you can get through this. It's okay to cry, but you also need to research. Knowledge is power—you need to know what you're facing.'

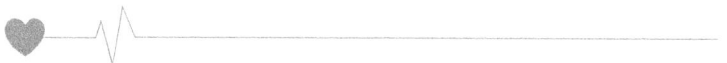

Her words were like a spark in the dark, and a flicker of determination began to ignite within me, pushing back against the suffocating despair. 'You're right,' I replied, wiping my tears with the back of my hand. 'I need to understand what this means for our baby. I can't let fear paralyse me.'

'I'm here for you,' Clara reassured me, her voice a steady pillar. 'You're going to be an incredible mum through all of this. I know it's hard right now, but you'll find a way. Just remember, you have me behind you. I'm always just a phone call away.'

Her words, so full of love and support, began to lift me up. 'Your baby is going to be fine,' she insisted with confidence, and even though it felt hard to believe, I found myself clinging to her words.

'He is a boy,' I said gently, remembering how the sonographer had mistakenly revealed the gender earlier in the scan.

'Yay! Another boy,' Clara replied, and a small laugh escaped her, even through the tears. 'You're going to fight for him, and that fight will make all the difference.'

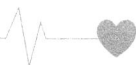

After hanging up with Clara, I knew I couldn't stop there. I had to reach out to the rest of my family. I dialled my sisters, Chloe, Cora, Olive and Iris. Each conversation felt like another heavy weight added to my shoulders, but it was also a reminder that I wasn't carrying it alone. Chloe, Cora, Olive and Iris each offered their love, encouragement and unique perspectives. Iris, who had a medical background, asked me more specific questions about the appointment. When I told her what the cardiologist had said, she assured me that she'd seen similar cases before and urged me to fight for my baby.

'Never consider termination,' she said firmly. 'Every situation is unique, and you'll find your strength, just like you always have.'

Cora, ever the pessimist, bluntly reminded me to consider every possibility and worst-case scenario. 'This journey will be tough,' she said, 'and you have to be prepared for anything. It won't be easy, but whatever you choose, make sure it's what's best for your family.'

Olive and Chloe were a bit more cautious, urging me to take things one step at a time. 'Don't rush any decisions,' Olive said. 'Do what feels right for you and your family. We're here for you, no matter what.'

With each call, I felt the weight of the situation settle a little more comfortably. It was a powerful reminder that I wasn't alone in this fight. My family, my friends would stand beside me, ready to shoulder the experience with me.

When I ended the call with my sisters and Clara, I looked over at Tee, who was still driving, his grip on the steering wheel tight. I took his hand, the simple act grounding me. 'No matter what,' I said, my voice barely above a whisper, 'we'll fight for our heart-baby.'

Tee nodded without hesitation. His eyes focused on the road, but his presence filled the car with a quiet strength. 'We will,' he said. The steadiness in his voice left no room for doubt.

By the time we arrived at Willow and Ethan's house, the sounds of our children's laughter as they played together filled the air. It was a strange contrast to the heaviness in our hearts—the joy and innocence of childhood were so at odds with the weight we carried. We tried to mask our emotions as best we could, but it was clear something was wrong.

Willow and Ethan greeted us at the door with warm embraces, their concern evident in their eyes. Willow had prepared dinner, but we declined, too overwhelmed to

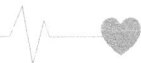

eat. She packed it up for us to take home, a small gesture that felt comforting in its simplicity. As we sat in their living room, the kids played happily in the background, oblivious to the storm that had descended upon us.

'How was the appointment?' Willow asked, her voice soft, her worry clearly written on her face.

I couldn't hold back the tears anymore, and I let them fall freely, the dam I'd been holding back cracking open. I shared the news with them, my voice shaking.

Willow immediately pulled me into a tight hug, her warmth surrounding me. She shared a story about her friend, a parent who had been told their child had a heart defect, but that child ended up not needing surgery. Her story, though different, gave me a flicker of hope. She reassured us both, telling Tee and me that they would support us no matter the decisions we made regarding the pregnancy.

After spending some time with them, we headed home. When we arrived home, Milo and Hugo continued to chat excitedly about their day. Tee prepared them for bed, and I sat in the living room, lost in thought. The world seemed to be moving in slow motion, each passing second heavy with the weight of the unknown.

Tee was upstairs, putting Milo and Hugo to bed, giving me a brief moment of solitude. I knew I needed to talk to Finn, my brother, the one person who always knew exactly how to ground me, especially when it came to matters like this. With his medical background, he had a way of making sense of things when everything felt like chaos. My hands slightly trembled as I reached for my phone, dialled his number and prayed for the comfort only he could provide.

'Hello, Ezy,' Finn answered, his voice calm and steady with the same reassuring tone I had heard all my life. 'What's going on? You don't sound like yourself.'

I took a shaky breath, my chest tight with the weight of the words I had to say. 'They diagnosed my baby with pulmonary atresia, VSD, and MAPCAs,' I said. The medical terms slipping off my tongue were foreign, but I had drilled them into my mind during the appointment. 'The doctor said he'll need surgery as soon as he's born, or he will not survive.'

A long pause hung in the air, and I could feel Finn processing the gravity of what I'd just shared. Then, his voice broke through the silence, strong and steady. 'Ezy,' he began, his tone gentle but firm, 'I know this is hard to hear, and I know it might seem overwhelming right now,

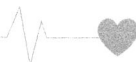

but your baby deserves a fighting chance. Please, please don't even think about considering the termination they mentioned. Every child deserves the chance to fight for their life, no matter the odds.

'I know it sounds like a lot right now, but the medical side of it... it's not always as bad as it seems. There's a lot of room for hope here. We'll get through this. We'll handle it. You'll handle it.'

His words washed over me like a wave of reassurance, grounding me in the moment. Despite the fear and uncertainty twisting in my gut, Finn's steady confidence reminded me that I wasn't alone in this, and I didn't have to navigate it on my own.

I closed my eyes, letting his words sink in. 'I feel so overwhelmed, Finn,' I whispered, my voice trembling. 'I'm just so scared.'

'Listen to me,' Finn said, his voice soft but resolute, 'you're stronger than you know. You've been through a lot already, and this is just another challenge you're going to face head-on. We'll be here every step of the way, helping you with the decisions you need to make.

'I'm not going anywhere. I'm here for you, always.'

Tears welled up in my eyes, but this time they were different. They weren't tears of fear—they were tears of gratitude. His words were like an anchor, pulling me out of the storm in my mind, reminding me that I had a solid support system behind me and that I wasn't alone in this.

'Thanks, Finn,' I said, my voice still shaking but stronger now. 'I needed to hear that.'

'I know you did,' he replied, his tone softening, a hint of warmth in his voice. 'Whatever you decide, just know I've got your back. Always. You've got a family that will do whatever it takes to support you and your baby, no matter what. We'll fight this together.'

We stayed on the phone for a few more minutes, talking through some of the medical details, but it was his unwavering confidence that kept me from drowning under the weight of it all. By the time we hung up, I felt a little lighter. Finn's words had given me the strength I needed to face the uncertainty ahead.

I took a deep breath, my hands still shaking but filled with a sense of purpose now. I knew the road ahead would be long and hard, but with Finn's support—and the support of everyone who loved me—I knew I wouldn't face it alone.

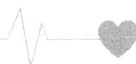

Once I hung up with Finn, I felt the need to talk to Ava. She had been a constant in my life, and I knew her presence would help me find a bit of peace. I had texted her earlier, sharing the news, and she rushed over to be with me. I opened the door to let her in and felt the warmth of her care before she even said a word.

We sat down on the couch, and Ava took my hands gently. 'Let's pray together,' she said, her voice gentle but confident, full of the kind of faith I desperately needed to feel.

I closed my eyes and let Ava's words wash over me. Her prayer was full of hope, strength and unwavering support, and I felt the weight of the world start to lift just a little, as though each prayer was a stitch in the fabric of the strength I needed to face this challenge.

When she finished, she looked at me, her eyes steady and filled with determination. 'No matter what decision you make, I'm here every step of the way. We're in this together.'

In that moment, I felt a warmth in my chest, a quiet, comforting fire fuelled by her faith and love.

Ava went home after about two hours, and I couldn't help but feel incredibly grateful for the support I had behind me.

Surrounded by the support and positive energy of my loved ones, I finally made the difficult decision to share the news with my elderly parents, who lived abroad. I hesitated at first, fearing it would upset them, especially knowing how deeply they felt things. I didn't want them to be burdened with such sadness, but as the encouragement around me grew, I realised it was important they knew, so I gathered my strength and called them. When I shared the news with my parents, their reactions were full of a love so deep and a concern so profound it almost made the distance between us disappear. My mum's voice, though shaken with emotion, was gentle but certain. She insisted, without hesitation, that I fight for my baby.

In the quiet that followed, she told me a story I had heard before but never with such weight. 'Ezy,' she began softly, 'you were just like your baby, born premature, significantly underweight. The doctors didn't think you would survive.'

Her words hit me like a wave, but then she said something that stopped my breath. 'Look at you today,' she continued, 'Your dad and I fought for you, and we

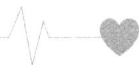

won. You must fight for your baby now. You must give him that chance.'

Tears welled in my eyes, each one a mix of sorrow. It was as if my mother had passed me a torch, handed over the very same courage she had drawn upon to fight for me all those years ago. At that moment, something deep inside me shifted, and I knew what I had to do. My baby deserved the same fight, the same unwavering love that had pulled me through, and I would fight, no matter the cost, just as my parents had fought for me.

The night stretched on, but I no longer felt quite so alone. With every conversation, every prayer, I felt the strength of the people who cared about me gathering around me like an invisible shield. It didn't take away the fear, but it did make it more manageable.

Later that night, Tee joined me in the living room, his presence steady and calming. He had just finished putting the kids to bed, and when he sat down beside me, I could see the concern on his face. He had been so quiet all evening, and I knew the weight of everything was bearing down on him, too.

'We'll figure this out, won't we?' he asked, his voice tinged with uncertainty, his eyes searching mine for some kind of reassurance.

I met his gaze and nodded, a newfound sense of determination rising within me. 'Yes, we will,' I replied decisively, my voice steady and strong despite the fear that still lurked. 'We have to fight for our heart-baby. No matter what it takes, we'll do whatever we can for him.'

Later that night, I sat at my laptop, determined to learn everything I could about pulmonary atresia. I wanted to understand the condition, the surgeries, the possible outcomes. I wasn't going to let fear take hold of me. I was going to arm myself with knowledge and use it as fuel to advocate for my child.

As I sifted through the articles and research, I came across posts from other parents who had gone through similar struggles. Their stories were painful, but filled with hope. Many of them had faced surgeries, complications and uncertainty, but they had come out on the other side stronger, more connected to their children than ever before. I found myself drawing strength from their words, a quiet but steady resolve building within me.

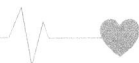

Clara's voice from our earlier call echoed in my mind: 'Knowledge is power.' She had been right. The more I learned, the less overwhelming the situation seemed. It wasn't easy, but I felt better equipped to navigate the storm.

I felt ready by the time I'd finished reading. The journey ahead would be long and difficult, but I was no longer afraid of the unknown. I had the strength of my family behind me, and I had the knowledge to face whatever came our way.

Tee and I sat together, side by side. For a moment, we didn't need to speak. We both knew that the path ahead was uncertain, but we also knew that, together, we would fight for our baby, no matter the challenges. And in every word of encouragement, every prayer, and every moment of support from our loved ones, we would find the strength to carry on.

CHAPTER 4

Testing the Unknown

After receiving an outpouring of support from our
loved ones, Tee and I felt a momentary lift, but the days
following the diagnosis stretched on endlessly. Each
hour felt like an uncharted journey, filled with questions
I couldn't answer. Why had this happened? What would
it mean for our baby's future? The world around me
seemed to move on as usual, but I felt trapped in a state
of suspended fear. Every little kick from my baby brought
a swirl of emotions, a glimmer of hope mixed with a deep
sense of sorrow. It was as if he was trying to reassure me
in his own way, yet I couldn't shake the feeling that we
were far from being out of the woods.

The cardiologist's appointment replayed in my mind
on an endless loop, leaving Tee and me feeling raw and

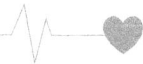

vulnerable. We knew we couldn't just wait—we needed answers to understand the full extent of our baby's condition. The doctor had suggested an amniocentesis, a procedure that could provide us with more information about potential chromosomal abnormalities.

Hearing the term 'amniocentesis' felt clinical, almost detached, like it belonged in a medical textbook, not in a conversation about our unborn child, but now, it had become central to our world. The decision to undergo the test weighed heavily on my heart—what if the results revealed even more challenges? The thought of receiving more bad news felt unbearable, yet I knew that having the information might give us some power, some semblance of control over the unknown. We needed to prepare ourselves for whatever lay ahead, no matter how daunting it seemed.

The choice was not an easy one. Tee and I sat together, holding hands in the quiet of our living room, wrestling with the decision.

'What do you think we should do?' Tee asked, his voice barely above a whisper. I could see the worry etched on his face, the same fear I felt mirrored in his eyes.

'I don't know,' I admitted, swallowing hard. 'I'm terrified of what the results might show, but... I also feel like we need to know. We need to be ready for whatever comes next.'

Tee nodded slowly, squeezing my hand. 'Whatever happens, we'll face it together, but if this test gives us a clearer picture, maybe we'll be able to make better decisions for him, you know?'

I took a deep breath, feeling the weight of his words. It was true—we couldn't make informed choices without knowing what we were up against. The fear of the unknown was overwhelming, but the thought of being unprepared was even worse.

'Okay,' I said finally, my voice steadier than I expected. 'Let's do it. Let's go ahead with the amniocentesis. I need to know what we're facing. We owe it to him to be as prepared as we can be.'

Tee pulled me into a tight embrace and rested his chin on my head. 'We'll get through this,' he murmured, 'one step at a time. No matter what, we're fighting for our baby.'

In that moment, I felt a flicker of strength return. It wasn't much, but it was enough to make the call and schedule

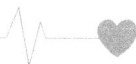

the test. We were stepping into the unknown, but we were doing it together, with our hearts set on giving our baby the best chance possible.

A few days later, a letter arrived in the mail, inviting us to the amniocentesis test. My hands shook as I opened it, and I felt my heart tighten as I read the details. This was real; there was no turning back now.

On the day of the appointment, Tee took the day off from work. We dropped Milo and Hugo off at school and nursery, trying to keep the morning routine as normal as possible for their sake, but I was a mess on the inside. I had barely slept the night before, my thoughts consumed by what lay ahead. Tee tried to reassure me with soft words and comforting touches, but I knew he was just as anxious as I was.

We arrived at the hospital in a tense silence. As we signed in at reception, the calm atmosphere of the place felt at odds with the storm inside me. The walls were painted a soothing shade of blue, but no colour could mask the tension that seemed to follow us wherever we went. The receptionist smiled kindly and directed us to sit in the waiting area until we were called. I glanced around the room, trying to distract myself from the gravity of what was about to happen. The other people in the room seemed lost in their own worlds, and I wondered if anyone else felt as broken as I did.

Tee held my hand tightly as we sat there, both lost in our thoughts. I leaned my head on his shoulder, seeking comfort in his presence, but the reality of our situation loomed large. My mind raced with what-ifs. What if the test revealed something more than just the heart defect? What if our baby had to face an even harder battle than we had anticipated? The uncertainty weighed on me like a stone, pressing down harder with each passing minute.

My name was finally called after what felt like forever. We stood up, our movements slow and heavy, as if we were walking through thick fog.

The nurse who greeted us was kind, her smile soft and genuine. She introduced herself and tried to put us at ease, chatting about inconsequential things to distract from the weight of the moment.

'You're doing great,' she reassured me as I lay down on the examination table. 'It's completely normal to feel nervous.' I nodded, grateful for her warmth, but the knot in my stomach wouldn't loosen.

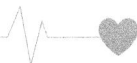

The doctor entered the room next, his demeanour professional and calm, though his presence only amplified my anxiety. He explained the procedure in a matter-of-fact tone, detailing how they would collect the amniotic fluid and test it for chromosomal abnormalities. His voice was steady, but I barely registered his words. My mind was miles ahead, already dreading what the results might show.

Tee leaned down and kissed my forehead, his lips soft against my skin. 'Everything will be fine,' he whispered, his voice filled with love and a hint of hope. I wanted to believe him, to hold onto that glimmer of optimism, but my heart was too full of fear to let it in.

The doctor prepped the ultrasound machine, and I watched the screen as he searched for our baby. My breath caught in my throat when I saw the tiny figure on the monitor, his little heartbeat fluttering away. Despite everything, seeing our baby brought a swell of love and protectiveness so strong it almost knocked the air out of me. That was our child, our little fighter, and no matter what happened, I would do everything in my power to keep him safe.

The doctor's voice broke the silence in the room. 'Your baby is moving quite a lot,' he said with a small smile. 'I'm having a hard time finding a good spot for the procedure.'

I laughed nervously, watching as our son squirmed and kicked on the screen, almost as if he were playing a game of hide and seek with the doctor. My heart twisted with a bittersweet feeling. The little life inside of me already had so much spirit, so much energy, even as we faced the unknown.

'We'll need to wait a bit,' the doctor said. 'Let's see if he settles down.'

I lay on the examination table, staring at the screen as the minutes ticked by. Time seemed to stretch out once again, each second filled with the anxious thrum of my heartbeat.

After about 20 minutes, our baby finally seemed to rest, his tiny form stilling on the screen. 'All right,' the doctor said, 'let's try again.'

This time, the doctor numbed the spot on my belly and prepared to insert the needle. My breath hitched as I saw the needle—it was longer than I had expected. Panic surged through me, my thoughts spiralling as I considered

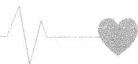

all the potential risks, but then I remembered Clara's words: 'Knowledge is power.' This was a necessary step.

I closed my eyes and took a deep breath, grounding myself in the belief that we were doing the right thing.

The doctor found the right spot, and I felt a sharp sting followed by deep pressure. It was over quickly, faster than I had anticipated, and the nurse was already applying a bandage to the site. 'See? You did it,' she said with a bright smile, her voice full of encouragement.

I managed a weak smile in return, though my mind was still reeling from the experience. The adrenaline was still coursing through my veins, making it hard to focus on anything but the weight of what had just happened.

'The hardest part is over,' the doctor said gently. 'Now, we just have to wait for the results. You should get a call in about two weeks.'

Two weeks. I thought about it, and it felt like an eternity. The wait stretched out before me like a dark tunnel with no promise of light at its end. The thought of spending the next 14 days trapped in a limbo of uncertainty made my heart ache. I couldn't shake the questions swirling in my mind: would the results bring more bad news? Would we have to face something even worse than we imagined?

As we left the hospital, I clung to the image of our baby on the ultrasound, the tiny heartbeat pulsing steadily. That image was my lifeline, a tangible reminder of hope amidst the fear.

In the car, the silence between Tee and I was heavy. I stared out the window, trying to calm the storm inside me, but the dread clung to me like a shadow, impossible to shake.

I pulled out my phone and saw that Ava had called. With a deep breath, I dialled her number, my hand faintly shaking as I hit the call button. Her voice was filled with concern the moment she answered.

'Hey, lovey, how did it go?' she asked, the worry clear in her tone.

'They took the sample,' I replied, forcing a note of optimism into my voice, though I knew she could hear the strain beneath it. 'Now, we just have to wait for the results.'

'Are you okay?' she asked gently.

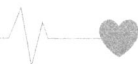

'I'm trying,' I admitted, the weight of it all pressing down on me. My voice faltered as the tears threatened to spill. 'I hate the waiting.'

'I know,' she said, 'but no matter what, I'm here for you. You're not alone."

Her reassurance was a small comfort, but it couldn't quell the storm of anxiety churning in my chest.

The days that followed felt as if they dragged on, each of them heavier than the last. I kept myself busy, diving into research, hoping for some clarity, but every search only pulled me deeper into a dark hole of fear. What if the results were bad? What if there were complications we hadn't prepared for?

During that time, I leaned heavily on the support of my family and friends, reaching out to them whenever the weight of my fears became too much to bear. My brother Finn's words echoed in my mind: 'Fight for your baby. You're stronger than you think.' My mother's comforting voice, sharing her experience with my birth, gave me the strength to keep going. Her words wrapped around me like a lifeline, reminding me that, even when the fear felt overwhelming, I wasn't alone.

Finally, after what felt like an endless moment the day arrived when I was supposed to hear back from the clinic. I was helping Milo and Hugo with their reading when my phone rang. My heart skipped a beat, leaping into my throat as I quickly answered.

'Hello, is this Lilian?' the voice on the other end asked, using my middle name.

'Yes,' I replied, my breath catching in my chest.

'I'm calling from the hospital with your amniocentesis results.'

My heart pounded as I waited for her to continue, each second stretching painfully out.

'I'm happy to inform you that the tests came back normal. No additional abnormalities were detected.'

Relief crashed over me like a seismic wave, and I collapsed onto the couch, tears streaming down my cheeks. I had been holding my breath for so long, and now, for the first time in weeks, I could finally breathe. Our baby still had a tough road ahead with his heart condition, but for the time being, I clung to the knowledge that we had been spared another devastating diagnosis.

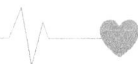

I thanked the woman on the phone repeatedly before hanging up, then turned to Tee, who was watching me with bated breath. 'It's good news,' I whispered, my voice breaking with emotion. 'The results are normal.'

Tee pulled me into his arms, holding me tightly as we both cried. It wasn't the end of our journey—not by a long shot—but in that moment, we allowed ourselves to feel hope, and for the first time in what felt like forever, it was enough.

That evening, I gathered with Tee and Milo and Hugo, taking a moment to reflect on our journey thus far. We talked about what the news meant for our family, sharing dreams of the future and the little moments we couldn't wait to experience together. We might not have had all the answers yet, but we did have each other, and that was enough to carry us forward into the unknown.

As I drifted off to sleep that night, I felt a sense of peace wash over me. Our journey was just beginning, but with hope, love and resilience as our guiding lights, I knew we would find our way.

CHAPTER 5

Decisions of the Heart

The days following the amniocentesis results felt like a whirlwind of emotions, a complex tapestry woven with threads of hope, fear, love and uncertainty. Tee and I received the news that our baby had no additional abnormalities, but there was still the overwhelming knowledge of the heart condition of pulmonary atresia with VSD and MAPCAs. As we processed this information, the magnitude of the decision before us loomed large. What did that mean for our pregnancy? For our family? Most importantly, how would we move forward?

The emotional landscape we found ourselves navigating was vast, marked by jagged peaks of anxiety and deep valleys of hope. We had so many questions and few definitive answers. Would our baby survive? What would

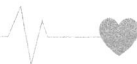

his quality of life be like? Could we handle the medical challenges ahead? How would this impact Milo and Hugo? Amidst the storms of our emotions, however, one truth anchored us: we wanted this baby. Whatever it took, we were determined to fight for that little life.

One evening, Tee and I sat together on the couch, the weight of our decision heavy in the air between us. The glow from a nearby living room lamp cast long shadows, mirroring the uncertainty that clouded our hearts. Tee was quiet, his brow creased in thought as he finally broke the silence.

'What do you think?' he asked, his voice filled with concern and uncertainty. 'Should we consider our options? Maybe get a second opinion to make sure we're well-informed?'

I took a deep breath, letting his words sink in. I couldn't help but recall the conversation I'd had with my sister Iris and my brother Finn, who both suggested that we seek a second opinion to be better informed. The reality of our situation was daunting, but one thing remained clear in my heart. 'I can't imagine not having this baby, Tee,' I replied, my voice trembling slightly but growing stronger with each word. 'I know it won't be easy, but I believe we can handle whatever comes our way. This child is a part of us, and I want to give him a chance.'

I paused, feeling the enormity of what we were deciding. 'But you're right: we should get a second opinion, just to know for sure what we're facing.'

Tee nodded slowly, his expression thoughtful as he processed my words. 'I agree,' he said finally, his voice steady. 'We're already in this together, and we'll figure out how to navigate the challenges. We have support. We're not in this alone.'

His words brought me a sense of comfort and unity. It was as if the weight on my shoulders had lightened just a little, knowing that we were a team, committed to each other and to our unborn child.

Still, I knew we couldn't face it alone. We needed the support of our family and friends, the people who had been there for us through life's other challenges. That night, I decided to reach out to my best friend, Clara. She had been a source of strength and wisdom for years, and I knew she would have the grounding perspective I needed.

I dialled her number, my hands gently quivering, I waited for her to pick up. When she answered, her warm voice immediately wrapped around me like a comforting blanket.

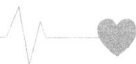

'Hey, how are you holding up?' she asked.

'I'm okay,' I said, though I knew it wasn't entirely true. 'I wanted to talk to you about the pregnancy… about the diagnosis. Tee and I are trying to make sense of everything, and I could really use your thoughts.'

'Of course,' she replied, 'I'm here. What's on your mind?'

I paused for a moment, the weight of my emotions pressing against my chest. 'Tee and I have been talking a lot about the future, about continuing the pregnancy. We know there will be challenges, but I can't imagine not giving our baby a chance. I just… I don't know if we're strong enough.'

There was a brief silence on the other end of the line as Clara absorbed my words. Then, her voice came through, filled with quiet confidence: 'You and Tee are two of the strongest people I know,' she said gently. 'I believe you can do this. It won't be easy, but the love you both have for this baby is clear, and you won't be alone. You have me, and you have your family. We'll all be here for you every step of the way.'

Her words resonated with me, filling the spaces of doubt with reassurance. Tears welled up in my eyes as

I whispered, 'Thank you, Clara. That means so much. I feel so overwhelmed, but knowing I have your support makes it a little easier.'

After hanging up, I felt a renewed sense of determination. Clara's words echoed in my mind as I reflected on the love surrounding us and the support we had from our family and friends. It gave me hope, reminding me that even in the darkest moments, we weren't alone.

Later that evening, I decided to gather my sisters—Chloe, Cora, Olive and Iris—for a video call, and their laughter and warmth filled the screen as soon as they appeared. We had always been close, and we talked about everything, from childhood memories to the latest family gossip, and for a moment, it felt as if the weight of the world had lifted.

The conversation eventually turned to my pregnancy. I shared my thoughts about continuing the pregnancy and the struggles Tee and I faced in making that decision. Their faces lit up with encouragement and love, giving me a sense of solidarity that I desperately needed.

'Whatever you decide, we'll be here," Iris said. The others echo her support, their eyes full of sincerity. 'You're not in this alone.'

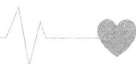

'I can't express how much that means to me,' I replied, my heart swelling with gratitude.

As the call ended, I felt lighter, my heart buoyed by the love of my sisters. We may have been separated by distance, but in that moment, they felt closer than ever.

Next, I reached out to my brother, Finn. He had always had a way with words, and I knew he would offer me a unique perspective.

When he picked up, his voice was filled with warmth. 'Hey, Ezy,' he greeted me. 'How are you feeling?'

'Honestly?' I hesitated, feeling the weight of my fears. 'I'm scared. We are keeping our baby, but the uncertainty… it's overwhelming.'

Finn was quiet for a moment, letting my words hang in the air before speaking. 'Remember, you've faced challenges before,' he said gently. 'You and Tee are strong, and you'll make the best decision for your family.

'No matter what, I'm here for you, and I'll support you every step of the way. Your baby deserves a chance to live, and that's what matters. I love you, and I'll be there with you all the way.' His unwavering support filled me with

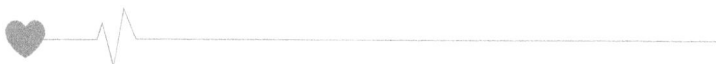

a renewed sense of strength. With each conversation, the weight of my fear began to lift, replaced by the collective strength of my family and friends. Their love enveloped me like a protective shield, guarding me against the uncertainty of the road ahead.

Feeling empowered, I reached out to my other best friend, Ava, who had always been a source of inspiration, her faith and resilience shining through even in the hardest of times. When she answered the phone, I heard the concern in her voice.

'Hey, how are you holding up?' she asked gently.

'I'm managing,' I replied, though the strain in my voice was unmistakable. 'I wanted to talk to you about the pregnancy, the diagnosis.

'Tee and I have decided to keep the baby, but I'm still grappling with the emotions. It feels like a lot.'

Ava's voice softened with understanding. 'I'm here for you, no matter what. Let's get together soon—I want to pray with you and support you in any way I can.'

Her words brought me comfort, and I felt deeply grateful to have such a strong support system. It wasn't just

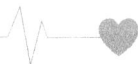

about deciding; it was about the love and encouragement surrounding me. With each conversation, I felt a little stronger, a little surer of the path ahead.

In the days that followed, Tee and I continued to talk about our decision. We considered the challenges: the potential hospital visits, the surgeries, the emotional toll of raising a child with a heart condition and our other two children. But even as we weighed the risks, we always came back to the same conclusion: we were committed to this little life. We would fight for our heart-baby together.

One evening, as we sat on the couch in a rare moment of calm, Tee turned to me, his eyes filled with love and anticipation. 'What do you envision for our baby?' he asked softly.

I smiled, my heart swelling at the thought. 'I want to see him play, to play with Milo and Hugo. I want to hear his laughter fill our home, watch him take his first steps, and see him off on his first day of school. I want to show him the world."

Tee nodded, his expression serious but full of determination. 'And we will. We'll be there through it all, no matter what challenges we face. We're a team, and we're going to give this baby every chance.'

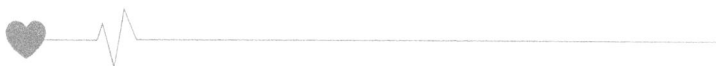

In that moment, I felt an overwhelming wave of love wash over me. The journey ahead was unpredictable, but our hearts were resolute. Bound by an unbreakable bond of family and love, we would face whatever came our way, hand in hand, ready to navigate the unknown.

That night, after Tee had fallen asleep, I sat down to write in my journal. I poured my heart onto the pages, writing about the love I already felt for our baby, the hope that filled me despite the uncertainty, and the unwavering support we had from our friends and family. Writing was cathartic, a way to process the swirling emotions inside me.

'Dear baby,' I wrote, 'even before you arrived, you brought so much love into our lives. You are cherished, and we are ready to fight for you. Whatever challenges lie ahead, we will face them together as a family. You are already so loved, and we can't wait to meet you.'

As I closed the journal, I felt a sense of peace wash over me. The decision had been made; Tee and I were all in. We would give our heart-baby every chance at life, no matter how hard the road ahead might be. With the love and support of our family and friends, we knew we could do it. The journey had just begun, but we were ready to face it head-on, filled with hope, faith, resilience and love.

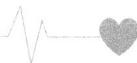

CHAPTER 6

Hope and Uncertainty

The days following our decision to continue the pregnancy were a delicate balance of hope and uncertainty. The news from the foetal cardiologist had settled into our lives like a weight we had to carry, yet we were determined to lighten it with the strength of our love and the unwavering support of those around us. Our future with our heart baby was uncertain, and we needed to know more. We craved clarity, an understanding of what was to come and how we might prepare for it. It was with this need for answers that we made the decision to seek a second opinion.

One quiet evening at home, Tee and I discussed the possibility of reaching out to another specialist. The house was still, the hum of the day fading as the children slept peacefully in their beds. The silence gave room for our

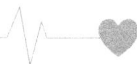

worries to surface, for the questions we had buried in the chaos of our daily lives to find their way to the surface.

'I know we've discussed it before,' Tee said, his voice steady as he leaned back against the couch, 'but I'm convinced it would be wise to get another perspective,' he searched my face as if looking for a sign of agreement. 'The more we know, the better prepared we'll be for whatever lies ahead.'

I nodded, feeling a mix of apprehension and determination. 'You're right,' 'It can't hurt to hear what another specialist has to say. If there's even a chance that surgery might not be needed right away, I want to explore it.'

We sat there for a moment, the weight of the conversation settling between us. This was our child's life we were talking about, the thought of surgery, especially so soon after birth, was terrifying, but there was also a spark of hope, a sliver of possibility that another opinion could provide a different path, one that might not involve immediate surgery.

With renewed purpose, we decided to reach out to a private cardiology clinic, one specialising in foetal cardiac scans. The process of scheduling an appointment was meticulous, filled with paperwork and phone calls, but we approached it with urgency, each step bringing us closer to the answers we sought, a flicker of light at the end of the long, dark tunnel.

The day of the appointment arrived, and with it came a whirlwind of emotions. I woke up that morning with a heavy feeling in my chest, knowing that by the end of the day, we would either have more hope or more worry.

The drive to the clinic was quiet, the weight of anticipation settling heavily in the car. I glanced over at Tee, his jaw set in determination as he focused on the road. I reached out, took his hand and squeezed it gently. 'We'll get through this together,' I said, my voice steady despite the nervous flutter in my stomach.

He glanced at me, his eyes softening for a moment. 'We will,' he replied. 'No matter what happens, we've got this.'

We walked through the clinic entrance; the sterile smell and bright lights all too familiar. We had been in and out of medical facilities so many times over the past few months that it almost felt like a second home, but this time, there was a hint of hope nestled amongst the anxiety. Maybe this doctor would tell us something different, something that would make the road ahead just a little bit easier.

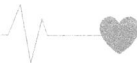

We checked in at the front desk and took a seat in the waiting area, surrounded by other families. Some looked relaxed, their faces lit with the glow of expectation, while others wore expressions of deep worry, their eyes heavy with uncertainty. It was a strange sort of comfort to sit among them, knowing that in this space, we were not alone in our fears.

The nurse called us back after what seemed like an endless wait. We followed her down a long corridor lined with colourful artwork, paintings of rainbows and flowers, likely designed to uplift the spirits of those who passed through. I couldn't help but feel a small sense of comfort in the environment. It was a place of healing, where hope and care intertwined.

We were led into the examination room where a sonographer was waiting, and I took a deep breath, reminding myself to stay calm. Soon, the cardiologist entered, her demeanour warm and reassuring. She introduced herself and sat with us, attentively listening as we recounted our journey thus far, our fears, our hopes and the weight of the decisions that lie ahead. I appreciated how she took her time, never rushing us, and it eased some of the tension that had been building up inside me.

After a thorough discussion, she prepared to perform an echocardiogram. 'Let's take a closer look at your baby's heart,' she said, her voice calm and soothing.

I laid back on the exam table, the cool gel was spread across my abdomen, and the familiar hum of the machine filled the room. As the images of our baby's heart appeared on the screen, I held my breath, my eyes fixed on the monitor.

The cardiologist moved the wand with precision, studying the heart closely. 'What we're looking for,' she explained, 'is how well the heart is functioning and whether there are any additional complications.'

Tee sat beside me, holding my hand tightly. I could feel his pulse, steady and strong as we waited together. The echocardiogram seemed to go on forever, each second stretching into what felt like an eternity. The silence in the room was heavy, broken only by the occasional click of the machine.

Finally, the cardiologist turned to us, her expression thoughtful. 'I'm happy to report that your baby's heart is functioning relatively well,' she said. 'While there are still concerns, as you are aware, your baby has pulmonary asteria, VSD and MACAPS, but it looks like surgery may not be needed immediately after birth.'

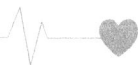

Relief washed over me so suddenly that I almost couldn't speak. I turned to Tee, and his eyes were wide with a mixture of hope and disbelief. 'Are you sure?' I asked, my voice barely above a whisper.

'Yes,' she reassured us. 'There are always risks, of course, but based on what I'm seeing here, we can take a wait-and-see approach. We'll monitor the baby closely after birth and develop a plan based on how things progress.'

The weight of uncertainty lifted just a little, replaced by cautious optimism. As we left the clinic, I felt lighter, as though a burden had been lifted from my shoulders.

We made our way back to the car, and I couldn't contain the smile that spread across my face. 'I can't believe it,' I said, my voice bubbling with excitement. 'We might not have to rush into surgery right away!'

Tee grinned at me, his relief palpable. 'This is great news! We can take it one step at a time.'

As we drove home, I found myself reflecting on the journey we had been on thus far. The uncertainty that had loomed so large now felt a little more manageable. For the first time in a long while, there was a glimmer of hope on the horizon.

When we arrived home, the atmosphere felt different, lighter, somehow. Milo and Hugo were buzzing with energy, their laughter filling the space as they played. I gathered them close, their little faces alight with curiosity as I shared the news about their sibling. 'Guess what?' I said, excitement bubbling in my voice. 'We have some good news about the baby! The doctors say we might not need to rush into surgery right away!'

Their eyes widened, and they erupted into cheers, their joy evident. 'Does that mean we can play with the baby soon?' Milo asked, his eyes sparkling with excitement.

I laughed and pulled them into a hug. 'Possibly, yes. It means we have more time to get ready to welcome the baby, and that's something to celebrate!"

That evening, as we sat around the dinner table, I looked at Tee and our children and felt an overwhelming sense of gratitude. The path ahead was still uncertain, but for now, we had a moment of peace. It was a chance to revel in the joy of being together as a family.

Later that night, after the kids had finally drifted off to sleep, Tee and I sat together on the couch, the quiet of the evening wrapping around us. We reflected on the

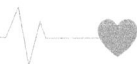

day, and the weight of everything finally started to feel a little lighter.

'I can't believe how much hope we have now,' Tee said softly, his voice filled with warmth and something deeper: an unmistakable sense of peace.

'Me, too,' I replied, leaning against him, feeling the strength of his presence. 'It won't be easy, but I feel like we're ready to face whatever comes our way.'

In the stillness of the moment, a thought came to me, one that felt like the right time to say aloud: 'Can we name him Lion?' I asked, my voice tinged with hope.

Tee turned to me, his eyes softening as he smiled. 'I can't think of a better name,' he replied, his voice steady with certainty. 'Our Lion.'

The significance of calling him Lion went beyond just a name—it became a symbol, one of strength, courage and resilience, qualities we hoped he'd embody throughout his life. Especially as we faced the challenges ahead, we wanted him to grow into someone who stood firm, just like the noble animal his name evoked. Lions represent power, fearlessness and a spirit that refuses to back down, traits we believed would guide him through adversity. It was a name that held not only the potential of his future but also the fierce love and protection we had for him at the time as we stood ready to fight for him as the guardians of his future. It would be a constant reminder that, no matter what we faced, we would do it together, and he would stand tall and strong, just like his namesake.

As we spoke, the darkness of uncertainty still lingered, but it no longer felt as overwhelming. It was there, yes, but now it was tempered by something brighter, the possibility of something better, the chance to navigate this journey together, hand in hand, with hope as our guiding light.

In the days that followed, I held onto that sense of hope. I found myself reaching out to other parents who had been through similar experiences, seeking comfort in their stories. Each conversation was a reminder that we were not alone on this journey. We had a community of support, a network of love that would carry us through.

The support from friends and family continued to uplift us; their words of encouragement a constant source of strength. 'You're going to be an amazing mom to this little one,' Iris told me during one of our phone calls. 'Just remember, no matter what happens, you've got us behind you.'

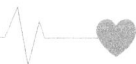

'I know,' I replied, my heart swelling with gratitude. 'I couldn't do this without all of you.'

As the pregnancy continued, I learned to live with both hope and uncertainty. I embraced the highs and lows, finding solace in the love that surrounded me. Each day brought us closer to meeting our heart-baby, and with that came a growing sense of strength and determination.

At night, as I lay in bed, my hand resting on my belly, I whispered words of love and encouragement to the little life growing inside me: 'You are so loved, little one. Whatever challenges lie ahead, we will face them together. You are a part of us, and we will fight for you, no matter what.'

In those quiet moments, I realised that this journey, with all its ups and downs, had already begun to shape me in ways I hadn't expected. It was teaching me the true meaning of resilience, the power of love and the importance of holding onto hope, even in the darkest of times.

CHAPTER 7

Balancing Act

Hope and uncertainty filled my days following the second opinion appointment regarding my baby's cardiac condition. While the relief of that consultation provided some comfort, the journey ahead still felt uncertain. Amidst countless hospital appointments and visits, I'd been juggling my studies along with the responsibility of caring for my two young children.

The sun rose each morning with a relentless brightness, its golden rays seeping through the thin blinds of my bedroom window, making it impossible to sleep any longer. It pierced through the glass, illuminating every corner of the room, but more than that, it penetrated the walls I'd carefully built around myself, exposing the fragility of my current reality. As I reluctantly opened my

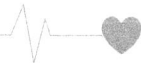

eyes, the weight of the day ahead immediately pressed on my chest. Each morning felt like the universe was nudging me to get up and face yet another day full of responsibilities that I was not sure I could juggle.

In the distance, I heard my children's lively chatter. Milo's commanding tone rang out, his words sharp and direct as he attempted to boss his younger brother around. Ever the playful one, Hugo responded with giggles, refusing to follow his brother's orders but enjoying the game nonetheless. Their voices had become the soundtrack to my life, moments of sibling rivalry punctuated by bursts of infectious laughter that should have filled me with joy but often weighed heavily on my already overburdened heart. It was not that I didn't love their noise, their chaos, their vibrancy; it's just that in those moments, the fluttering in my stomach—a constant reminder of my pregnancy—told me that I was carrying the weight of not just three children, but three separate worlds that relied on me.

I struggled to pull myself out of bed, the physical weight of my growing belly having added to the emotional load I'd been carrying for months. Every step felt heavier, slower, more deliberate. I moved towards the bathroom, my hand instinctively resting on my swollen belly as if to steady myself both physically and mentally. The cold tiles beneath my feet woke me up a little more, and I turned on the shower, hoping that the rush of water would cleanse not just my body but my mind, too. There was so much to do that day. There was always so much to do.

Hugo burst into the bathroom unannounced, his curly hair sticking up in all directions, his wide grin making it impossible to be upset with him. 'Mummy! he chirped, triumphantly holding up one of his toy cars. '*Vroom, vroom!*' His innocence was disarming. I smiled despite myself and ran my hand over his head, wishing I could hold onto his carefree nature, but reality pulled me back.

'Milo… Hugo… breakfast time!' I called out as I headed towards the kitchen, my hand absentmindedly rubbing my lower back. The aches and pains of pregnancy seemed to worsen every day, a cruel reminder that my third pregnancy was taking more out of me than the others, but there was no time to dwell on it. I had to keep moving. There was breakfast to be made, school drop-offs to manage, a full day of my social work placement to get through, and then, of course, the hospital appointment that loomed over me like a dark cloud.

As I whipped up pancakes for Milo, who'd been adamant when requesting them all morning, I felt a rush of anxiety wash over me. It was not the usual frantic morning

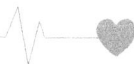

routine—the hospital appointment was later that day, the foetal cardiology appointment that would determine how my baby's heart was doing. My heart raced at the thought of it. Would that bring more bad news, or would it be a small reprieve, something to hold onto for a while longer?

'Mum, where's the syrup?' Milo's voice snapped me out of my thoughts; his brow wizened in frustration as he inspected his pancake plate.

I quickly handed him the syrup bottle and offered him a reassuring smile, though inside, I felt far from calm. 'Here you go, love. Eat up. We don't want to be late for school.'

The clatter of forks against plates, the chatter about their day ahead, the requests for more milk—it all blended together into a familiar, comforting rhythm, but beneath the surface, my mind was elsewhere. I was thinking about the echocardiogram later that day, the scan that would show my baby's tiny heart beating inside me, fragile and vulnerable, just like me.

After breakfast, I rushed the children into their clothes, dodging the inevitable last-minute requests. Milo, ever the perfectionist, insisted on wearing his favourite vest,

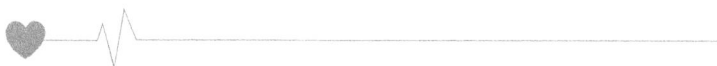

while Hugo refused to leave without his toy truck. The clock was ticking, and my patience was wearing thin. 'Come on, guys! We have to go!' I shouted, already feeling as if I'd fallen behind.

Once they were finally buckled into their car seats, I sat in the driver's seat for a moment and took a deep breath. My phone buzzed with a calendar reminder; the words 'Foetal Cardiologist, 2:00 p.m.' flashed across the screen.

I stared at the notification, feeling the now-familiar pang of fear in my stomach. It was not just the physical discomfort of the pregnancy that had been weighing on me but the emotional toll of carrying a child whose future felt so uncertain. Every doctor's appointment, every scan, brought with it the possibility of more bad news. I tried to steel myself, remind myself that I'd made it that far, that I could do it, that I had to do it.

The school drop-off was the usual frenzy of backpacks, lunch boxes and goodbye hugs. Milo skipped off without a second thought, but Hugo clung to me a little longer. 'Love you, Mummy,' he whispered, his small arms wrapped tightly around my neck. I closed my eyes for a moment, soaking in his warmth before reluctantly letting him go. There was always a part of me that felt guilty for leaving them, for not being more present, but there

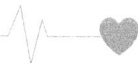

was also the part of me that knew I had to keep pushing forward for them and for the baby growing inside me.

As I drove to my social work placement, my thoughts drifted back to the upcoming appointment. What would the doctor say this time? Would there be more complications? Would we finally get more good news? The questions swirled around in my head, and I felt that familiar lump in my throat, but I couldn't let myself cry, not then, not yet.

Upon arriving at my placement, I was greeted with the warmth and routine I'd come to rely on, but on that day, the weight of my other responsibilities—not just as a mother but as a student—felt more intense. The deadlines loomed large: essays that needed to be written, assessments due at the end of the week, and the ever-present pressure of my placement itself. Balancing all of that with my pregnancy felt like an impossible feat. The deadlines came in waves: clinical reflections, assessments and academic commitments for my second-year social work course. Each deadline bore down on me like another layer of weight that I was constantly trying to hold up while still giving everything I had to my growing baby and children.

Somehow, I managed to push through. My placement supervisor was understanding, but the work didn't let

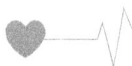

up. Reports, case studies and assessments waited for no one, not even an overwhelmed pregnant mother. In the back of my mind, I knew I'd have to explain the latest developments in my pregnancy and probably take more time off soon. I could only hope that by the time the baby arrived, I'd managed to keep everything afloat, even if just barely.

As the day wore on, I was consumed by thoughts of the appointment. Finally, when 2:00 p.m. rolled around, I was sitting in the sterile, brightly lit waiting room of the hospital, surrounded by other expectant mothers and their partners. Some looked calm as they chatted happily about baby names and nursery plans. Others, like me, sat in tense silence, clutching their phones or holding their partners' hands a little too tightly. I sit alone, my phone buzzing with messages from friends and family offering their love and support, but it didn't make the waiting any easier.

When my name was finally called, I followed the nurse into the exam room, my heart pounding in my chest. The room was cold, and the smell of antiseptic stung my nose. I lay back on the examination table, my shirt pulled up to expose my swollen belly. The gel was cold against my skin, and I flinched as the technician pressed the ultrasound wand against my abdomen.

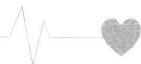

The screen flickered to life, showing the familiar black-and-white image of my baby. I held my breath as the technician moved the wand around, focusing in on the tiny beating heart. I heard the *whoosh-whoosh* of the blood flow, the rhythmic pulsing of life inside of me. I wanted to ask questions, but my throat felt tight, and I couldn't bring myself to speak.

The doctor entered the room, his expression neutral, giving nothing away. He reviewed the images on the screen, his brow lined in concentration. My heart raced as I waited for him to speak, my hands clenched tightly in my lap.

Finally, he looked at me, his expression softening just slightly. 'Your baby's heart is stable for now,' he said, his voice calm and measured. 'We'll continue to monitor closely, but there's no immediate concern. We'd like to induce you at full term as long as things stay stable.'

Relief flooded through me, and I exhaled a breath I didn't realise I was holding. There was no need for immediate intervention and no emergency surgeries. The thought of inducing labour at full term felt like a gift, something normal amidst all the chaos. It was not perfect, but it was something.

It was enough for now.

The rest of the day passed in a blur. I picked the kids up from school, helped with homework, cooked dinner, and went through the usual bedtime routines, but as I sat in the quiet of the evening with the children finally asleep, the weight of the day still pressed down on me. My mind replayed the cardiologist's words, 'No immediate concern,' over and over, clinging to them like a lifeline, but even in the relief, there was an underlying tension, an awareness that we were not out of the woods yet. The baby's heart was stable for now, but what about tomorrow? Next week? The weeks leading up to full term feel like an eternity when you're living under the shadow of uncertainty.

I sat at the kitchen table, the soft glow of the overhead light casting long shadows across the room. My textbooks and laptop were spread out in front of me, a reminder that the demands of my university deadlines weren't going anywhere. My second-year social work coursework had become a delicate balancing act. I'd been working on various assessments, each with its own looming deadline. There were case studies to analyse, reflections on practice to write, and assessments to prepare for, all while navigating the emotional rollercoaster of my pregnancy.

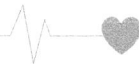

That night, I had to submit a reflective journal for my placement. My mind was foggy with fatigue, but I knew I couldn't afford to fall behind. I opened my laptop, fingers hovering over the keyboard, trying to focus on the task at hand. The words didn't come easily. My thoughts drifted back to the hospital, to the steady *whoosh-whoosh* of my baby's heartbeat, and the relief I felt in that fleeting moment.

I pulled myself back to the present. There was no time to get lost in my thoughts. My placement demanded my full attention. As a second-year social work student, I was learning how to balance empathy with professionalism, how to offer support to others while keeping my own emotions in check, but that balance had been harder to maintain lately. How could I help others when my own world felt so fragile?

The clock ticked on, and finally, I managed to type out a few coherent paragraphs. It was not my best work, but it'd have to do for now. I submitted the assignment and closed my laptop, feeling a wave of exhaustion wash over me.

Just as I was about to head to bed, my phone buzzed with a message from my placement supervisor. She'd been incredibly understanding about my situation, offering support and flexibility whenever I needed it, but that night's message was a reminder of the upcoming assessments I needed to complete, deadlines I couldn't afford to miss if I wanted to stay on track for graduation.

I sighed and ran a hand through my hair. The weight of everything felt so heavy that night. The endless deadlines, the constant hospital appointments, the fear for my baby's health and the pressure to be a good mother to Milo and Hugo—it was all too much sometimes, yet I knew I had to keep going. There was no other choice.

Lying in bed later that night, I rested my hand on my belly, feeling the gentle movements of my baby. Each kick was a reminder that life was still growing inside of me, that despite all the uncertainty, there was hope. The cardiologist's words replayed in my mind: 'We'll monitor you closely, but there's no immediate concern.' It was enough for the time being. It had to be.

As I drifted off to sleep, I told myself that tomorrow was another day. Another day to juggle my children, my placement, my university work and my baby's health. Another day to fight for my family and my future. The journey was far from over, but on that night, I allowed myself a small moment of peace because, sometimes, that's all we can ask for.

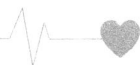

CHAPTER 8

The Baby Shower Celebration

The relief from Lion's amniocentesis test and ultrasound scan results hung in the air like the sweet scent of flowers filling our home as we prepared for the day we had been eagerly anticipating for weeks. After all the fear, the waiting, and the uncertainty, we finally had a reason to celebrate. That day was about joy, pure and simple. It wasn't just about the impending arrival of our baby; it was a chance to come together with family and friends and bask in the happiness that had been elusive in our journey so far.

We had endured emotional highs and lows, moments of hope and fear, but that day was different. That day

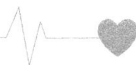

was about celebrating the joy we had fought so hard to hold onto.

The baby shower wasn't just a celebration of new life—it was a tribute to resilience, to battles fought and won and to the incredible support that had surrounded us every step of the way. After receiving the amniocentesis results and learning that Lion didn't need any further tests, Tee and I felt a wave of relief wash over us. For the first time in months, we could fully embrace the excitement of meeting our baby, free from the constant shadow of worry. It was a moment to let go of the fear that had lingered and allow us to truly celebrate.

As the day of the baby shower approached, excitement filled the air. Tee and I took on the task of decorating for the baby shower with excitement as we both shared a love for creating beautiful spaces. We wanted the decorations to reflect not just the joy of welcoming our baby boy but also the resilience and love that had carried us through the difficult months of pregnancy. Every little detail was carefully thought out, from the colours to the layout, as we knew that day would be a special one.

Together, we transformed the living room into a space that felt both intimate and celebratory. We decided on soft pastel shades of blue and yellow, symbolising both the calm and happiness we longed for. Tee worked on hanging the large 'Welcome Baby' banner at the entrance while I arranged delicate streamers that added a playful touch to the room. We also placed bouquets of fresh flowers on the tables, their delicate fragrance weaving through the house and creating a warm, welcoming atmosphere.

The balloons were perhaps one of our favourite elements. Tee meticulously arranged clusters of them around the room, creating a sense of movement and lightness, while I added personalised touches like tiny name tags and soft ribbons to tie everything together. The centrepiece, however, was the dessert table, a spread of sweets and finger foods we'd decorated with intricate details. Every cupcake, cookie and piece of cake was arranged with care, as if it represented the love and hope we had for Lion's future.

As we stepped back to admire the final look, a wave of pride washed over us. This wasn't just a baby shower — it reflected our journey, our partnership and the joy we had finally allowed ourselves to feel. It was our way of embracing this new chapter together, celebrating not just the arrival of our baby but the strength and unity we had found along the way.

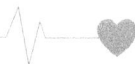

My best friend, Ava, had taken charge of the entire event, telling me, 'You don't need to worry about anything. This is your time to relax.' She had been a steadfast source of strength and positivity throughout our journey, always reminding me to focus on the brighter moments. True to her word, she and my other close friends handled every detail, from the games to the food. The love that poured into planning that day made it even more special.

We also decided to use the baby shower to share a long-awaited surprise: a gender reveal for the family members who didn't already know. While I had told my closest circle about our baby boy, the broader family was still in the dark, and we were excited to reveal Lion's gender in a way that would bring joy and laughter to everyone. The celebration wasn't just about our baby's arrival but about giving everyone—ourselves included—a reason to smile after such a turbulent journey.

The morning of the baby shower was nothing short of magical. Our home, now a vibrant and festive space, radiated warmth and love. But then, my outfit for the shower arrived late, throwing me into a mini panic.

I called my close friend, Sarah, who, without hesitation, rushed over to help me search through my wardrobe. After rummaging through countless options, we decided to make a quick trip to the mall. Sarah kept me calm, her light-hearted jokes helped to soothe my anxiety.

After what felt like endless store visits, we finally found the perfect outfit. 'This is my gift to you,' Sarah said, smiling. Her generosity warmed my heart, and I hugged her, grateful for her presence not just in that moment but throughout our entire journey. We hurried home, knowing that the guests would be arriving soon.

When people started arriving, the atmosphere shifted from anticipation to pure joy. Family and friends greeted us with tight hugs, their faces alight with excitement. Their laughter was infectious, and I found myself revelling in the rare, joyous occasion.

Ava had truly outdone herself with the baby shower games, ensuring that every moment of the day was filled with joy, laughter, and fun. She knew exactly how to lift everyone's spirits and make the event memorable. One of the first games, 'Guess the Bump Size', had everyone eagerly lining up to take their best guess. Each guest was given a piece of string and had to cut it to the length they thought matched the size of my baby bump. The room erupted with laughter as people measured their strings against my belly, with guesses ranging from comically short to absurdly long. Some even wrapped their string

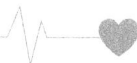

around themselves multiple times, convinced they had it right! The creative and wildly inaccurate predictions not only had everyone in stitches but served as the perfect icebreaker. It instantly lightened the mood and helped everyone relax, setting the tone for the rest of the afternoon.

Another game, the 'Diaper Relay,' had everyone in fits of laughter, really bringing the room to life. Teams were tasked with creating makeshift diapers out of tissue paper, using one person from their team as the 'baby'. The sight of grown adults frantically wrapping each other in fragile tissue and trying to secure their makeshift diapers without tearing them was hilarious. As the tissue inevitably ripped and participants fumbled through the challenge, the room filled with uncontrollable laughter. It was exactly what we all needed: a moment to let go of our worries, enjoy each other's company, and simply be present in the joy of the day.

The games weren't just a source of fun. The room buzzed with happiness, and in those moments, the weight of the past months felt a little lighter. Ava had turned what could have been just another event into a celebration of love, community and, most importantly, laughter.

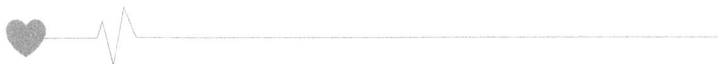

The highlight of the day was, of course, the gender reveal. We chose to share the news in a fun and heartwarming way: with a cake. Ava handed Tee and me a knife, and together, we stood in front of our friends and family, ready to reveal our secret. The room fell silent, the anticipation building as we cut into the cake. When the blue sponge was revealed, the room erupted into cheers.

'It's a boy!' I exclaimed, my voice thick with emotion. Tears filled my eyes as Milo and Hugo, jumped up and down in excitement, their joy matching mine.

That moment, surrounded by love and support, was one I will never forget. After months of uncertainty, fear, and difficult decisions, we had finally arrived at a place of pure happiness. It was as if a weight had been lifted, and for the first time in a long time, I felt nothing but joy.

As the afternoon wore on, the celebration continued with laughter, stories, and heartfelt conversations as everyone shared in the happiness of the moment. We opened the gifts that our friends and family had lovingly chosen for Lion, each tiny onesie and soft blanket a tangible reminder of the lover that had carried us through our journey. Every gift was a symbol of hope, and I couldn't help but feel overwhelmed by gratitude.

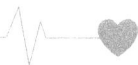

At one point during the celebration, I took a moment to step back and observe the scene unfolding before me. The room was alive with laughter and conversation, the air filled with the warmth of friendship and family. Milo and Hugo played with balloons while Tee was deep in conversation with his closest friends. It was a scene I couldn't have imagined only a few months earlier. The fear that had once seemed so overwhelming now felt like a distant memory, replaced by the peace and contentment of the joyful occasion.

As the day ended, Ava raised a glass to propose a toast. 'To Lion,' she said, her voice filled with emotion. 'To the miracle of life and to the strength of this incredible family.' Her words resonated deeply with me, and as we raised our glasses, I felt a deep sense of connection and gratitude. This was more than just a celebration of our baby; it was a celebration of resilience, of love and of the strength we had found in each other through the most challenging times.

That evening, as the guests began to leave and the house quieted down, I reflected on the day. The baby shower had been about so much more than the upcoming birth of our son. It was a reminder that we had already won countless battles, that we had come through the storm and emerged stronger on the other side. Our journey wasn't over, but that day, filled with laughter, love and hope, was a testament to the power of community and resilience.

As I stood in the now-empty living room surrounded by balloons and leftover cake, I felt ready—ready to meet our baby boy, ready to face whatever challenges might lie ahead, and ready to embrace the future with an open heart.

The road ahead was still unknown, but with the love and support of those around me, I knew we could face anything. We had already come so far, and I was confident that whatever came next, we would continue to walk our journey with hope and strength.

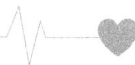

CHAPTER 9

A Tumultuous Birth

In the months following Lion's diagnosis, everything had shifted. While my antenatal care continued at our local hospital, the reality of his heart condition meant his birth would be unlike any I had imagined. As his diagnosis became more complex, my care was eventually transferred to a different hospital, where a specialized team from the same trust would take over Lion's specialised cardiac care. This would also be where I would deliver him. Knowing the seriousness of his condition, the medical team decided it was best to induce labour under controlled circumstances so his care could begin immediately after birth.

When the induction was scheduled, it marked the start of what would become an emotionally and physically

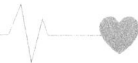

exhausting process. Lion's arrival meant that we would be surrounded by uncertainty and the presence of specialists ready to assess his condition the moment he was born. Despite the cloud of fear that hung over us, there was a deep sense of trust in the medical team guiding us through the unknown.

At last, the day of my induction arrived at 39 weeks and one day. It felt like an eternity had passed since the 20-week scan had cast a shadow over my pregnancy. Our journey had been a whirlwind of appointments, anxiety and endless prayers, but now, the moment we had longed for was finally here — the moment I would meet my baby, Lion. I tried to steady myself, clinging to hope despite the uncertainty that lay ahead. The doctors had prepared us for potential complications, but the road forward was still a mystery.

Finn had flown in from abroad to care for our other children, allowing Tee and me to focus solely on Lion's birth without the added stress of worrying about our other kids. As we made our way to the hospital, our nerves were masked by a quiet anticipation. Each step felt heavy, not just from the physical toll of the pregnancy but from the emotional weight we carried. The hospital walls echoed with the questions swirling in my mind: Would Lion be okay? What if things didn't go as planned? From early on in the pregnancy, I learned to expect the unexpected.

'Tee, I'm scared,' I whispered, gripping his hand as the induction began. His presence was steady, his touch grounding me amidst the wave of uncertainty. Throughout the pregnancy, he had been my rock, always strong when I felt as if I might drift away. Now, as the contractions began to slowly build, his hand in mine was a silent promise that we were in this together.

The room around us was calm, deceptively so, as if unaware of the storm slowly looming inside me. I lay there feeling each contraction roll through my body like waves gathering strength, but despite the growing intensity, nothing seemed to be happening. My body, stubborn and slow to respond, left us in a frustrating limbo. Time stretched, hours turning into a blur of discomfort that sharpened into pain.

'You're doing great,' Tee said softly, his voice a lifeline through the haze. His eyes, full of quiet strength, met mine, and in that moment, words weren't necessary. We were scared, both of us, His grip tightened as the pain intensified, but his presence never wavered.

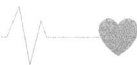

'Just breathe,' he whispered, his breath close to my ear. 'You've got this.'

I wanted to believe him, but my body refused to cooperate. With each passing hour, I sensed the tension in the room as the doctors exchanged glances.

After 48 hours, the doctors decided to break my waters, hoping to speed things along. The procedure was quick, just a sharp pressure followed by an empty rush. Still, there was no real progress. The contractions became heavier, each one more unbearable than the last, and the labour dragged on, slow and maddening.

'Tee,' I gasped during a particularly intense contraction, 'what if... what if this doesn't go the way we hoped?'

His thumb brushed the back of my hand, and for a moment, the chaos of the room faded. 'No matter what happens, we're going to get through this. Just focus on the next breath.'

Time began to lose meaning. The hours blurred into each other as pain consumed me, but underneath the pain was a growing dread. I knew that once our baby, Lion, had arrived, there wouldn't be that instant moment of bonding I had experienced with my other children. There would

be no first cuddle, no immediate skin-to-skin contact. The specialists would be waiting to whisk him away for the urgent care he needed.

I had mentally prepared myself for this, but as the moment inched closer, the ache in my chest grew. I wasn't ready to let go so soon after meeting him.

At last, after what seemed like a lifetime, the end was near. I could feel Lion descending, the unmistakable pressure signalling that our baby was about to enter the world. A surge of relief mixed with heartbreak rushed over me. I wanted to hold him, to feel his tiny body against mine, but I knew the reality that awaited us. With one final push, Lion entered the world at 39 weeks and three days.

The delivery room, which had felt almost intimate only moments earlier, was suddenly filled with a swarm of healthcare professionals. Cardiologists, Paediatricians, midwives, and Neonatal Intensive Care Unit (NICU) nurses all stood in tense readiness, their eyes fixed on Lion, each one braced for whatever his fragile heart might need. The air was thick with unspoken tension as if every breath in the room was collectively held, waiting for that first sign—any sign—that he was okay.

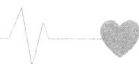

The room erupted into movement, a flurry of medical urgency I could barely process. My heartbeat thundered in my ears, drowning out the voices of doctors and nurses moving with precision and purpose around Lion.

Fear clenched my chest, tightening with every second. Would his tiny heart be strong enough? Would he need immediate intervention? These questions, unspoken but heavy, filled the air as the team closed in around him, their faces tense, bracing for the worst.

For months, this moment had loomed over us like a storm cloud. The uncertainty of Lion's condition had hung in the background, shaping every decision, every preparation. Now, it was here; this was the moment we had been dreading and hoping for all at once.

And then, as if the universe itself shifted. Something miraculous happened: despite all the fear, the anxiety, the months of preparation for an emergency, Lion didn't need the intense intervention everyone had braced for. His heart—though imperfect—was beating on its own. A stunned silence fell over the room. The frenetic energy dissolved, and for a moment, time seemed to stop.

'His heart is strong enough,' someone whispered, but the words barely registered.

Tears welled in my eyes as they placed him in my arms. I could hardly believe it. His small, warm body pressed against my chest, fragile but alive, so alive. His heartbeat—a steady, miraculous rhythm—pulsed softly against me, anchoring me to the breathtaking moment. I held him close, the tears spilling over as I whispered, 'You're here. You're really here.'

I had waited so long for the chance to hold him, to feel his heart beating next to mine. Against all odds, he was here, and his heart was strong enough. I looked at Tee, who stood beside me, tears in his eyes, too. Neither of us said a word; we didn't need to. Our son was here. Our miracle was in my arms, and nothing in the world could take that moment away from us.

But just as quickly as the moment arrived, it was taken away. The doctors moved swiftly in, gently taking Lion from my arms to rush him to the NICU for observation. Tee followed closely behind them, his worried gaze never leaving our son. And just like that, I was alone. The room, once so full of people and purpose, now felt achingly empty. I had known that would happen—I had prepared myself for it—but no amount of preparation could have softened the sting of our separation. With my other children, I had held them for hours, breastfed them, whispered sweet words in their ears as we bonded

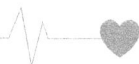

in those first precious moments of life, but now, my arms were empty, and my heart ached for Lion in a way words couldn't articulate.

I barely had time to process that sense of loss before everything changed. My body, which had endured the exhaustion of labour, now seemed to give way under the weight of it all. I began to feel strange—light-headed, dizzy—as if the ground beneath me was slipping away. The room spun, and a cold, eerie sensation crept through my body. Something was wrong, horribly wrong. I remember calling weakly out to the nurse, my voice barely above a whisper. She had been by my side through the entire process, her presence a constant source of calm, but now, her face tightened with concern. Without hesitation, she slammed the emergency button, and within seconds, the room filled with a rush of doctors, their urgency confirming my worst fears. Before I could fully grasp what was happening, I felt blood pouring out of me, hot and fast, draining the life from my body.

The nurse stayed beside me, still holding my hand, but her reassuring grip couldn't hide the seriousness in her eyes. I heard snippets of conversation as I drifted in and out of consciousness. The word 'haemorrhage' floated through the air like a dark cloud, and I felt my body grow lighter, weightless, as the blood loss took its toll. I struggled to stay awake, my vision fading. The last thing I saw was a blur of medical professionals hovering over me, their faces smeared by my fading vision before everything went black.

When I woke up, I was in a different room, groggy and weak. Machines beeped softly around me, and I realised I was on oxygen. My body felt heavy, unresponsive, and as I lay there, I overheard the healthcare professionals talking in hushed tones. The word 'hysterectomy' cut through the fog in my mind like a knife. My heart sank. They were talking about removing my uterus if they couldn't stop the bleeding.

Tee was still in the NICU with Lion. He had no idea what was happening, and I was completely alone, clinging to a fragile thread of awareness. They were preparing to take me into surgery, and fear gripped my soul. Would I survive this? Would I see Tee and my three children again? My mind raced, spinning through a whirlwind of terrifying thoughts as I floated in and out of consciousness.

Barely conscious, I whispered a prayer, 'God, please save me. I have three children who need me. Please give me the strength to survive this.' The fear of leaving my children motherless weighed so heavily on me that it felt as if my heart would break.

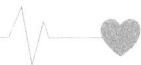

The doctors explained the situation: they would have no choice but to remove my uterus if they couldn't control the bleeding. I was too weak to talk. I had no choice but to trust them. With what little strength I had left, I whispered, 'Do whatever you need to do to save my life. I have three children.' My voice was barely audible, but I knew they'd heard me.

I signed the paperwork with trembling hands, the pen slipping through my fingers as I tried to focus, then I drifted back into unconsciousness, unsure of what the outcome would be.

When I finally woke again, the first thing I realised was that I was still alive. The bleeding was under control, and they managed to save my uterus. Relief washed over me, but I felt like a shell of myself, weak, exhausted, and emotionally drained. The nurses were incredible. Their warmth and professionalism were constant, guiding me through every stage of recovery with care and compassion. They had been there through the labour, through the birth, through the haemorrhage, and now, they were by my side as I began to heal. I couldn't have asked for a better team to carry me through the storm.

Hours later, Tee returned to my side, his face etched with worry, but when he saw me awake, the relief in his eyes was unmistakable. He told me that Lion was stable, and although we had a long road ahead, our little fighter was doing well. Hearing those words breathed life into me. We had both been so close to the edge, but we had made it. We were both alive.

The next 24 hours were a blur of recovery. Physically, I was drained, barely able to move. Emotionally, I felt completely raw, haunted by the trauma of nearly losing my life. The fear of leaving my children without their mother still gnawed at me, lingering in my heart, but what hurt the most was the separation from Lion. I ached to hold him, to bond with him the way I had with my other children. Instead, I lay in a hospital bed, alone, while Lion remained in the NICU, surrounded by machines and doctors.

I couldn't stop thinking about everything we had been through. The birth was nothing like I had imagined. With my other children, there had been no NICU, no complications, no brushes with death, but with Lion, everything about this experience had been unique from the very beginning. I was barely able to hold him before he was taken away. The bond I longed for, the closeness I expected, was delayed, and the emotional weight of that separation, of watching my baby being whisked away while I lay helpless, was almost too much to bear.

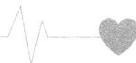

But through it all, I held onto hope. We had both survived, and I knew that soon, I would be able to hold Lion again. We had made it through the darkest moment, and now, all I could do was focus on healing for myself and for him.

During my recovery, as I lay there physically and emotionally drained, I found myself seeking something — anything — that would offer comfort or guidance. Desperate for answers, I turned to social media. I typed in Lion's heart condition and scrolled through countless posts from other parents who had walked the same difficult path. Each post felt like a window into a world where other families had also faced the terrifying uncertainty I was now living through.

That was when I stumbled upon a post from a mother whose child had been diagnosed with similar condition as Lion. Her words seemed to jump off the screen, radiating strength and resilience. Without hesitation, I reached out to her, not really expecting a response, but to my surprise, she replied almost immediately. Her message felt like a lifeline.

She shared her own harrowing journey, telling me about the surgeries, the hospital stays, and the countless sleepless nights. She spoke about advocating fiercely for her child, battling through moments of doubt and fear. Her story

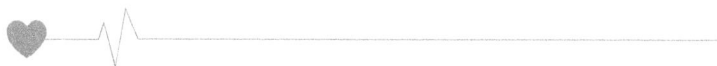

mirrored my own, and her unwavering determination to fight for her son struck a chord deep within me. 'Always fight for Lion,' she urged. 'No matter what, you're his voice, his protector. You've got this.'

Hearing those words breathed life into me, igniting a renewed sense of purpose. For the first time since Lion's birth, I felt a flicker of strength returning. I wasn't alone. There were other mothers out there—warriors—who had fought the same battles, and they had emerged stronger on the other side. If they could do it, so could I.

As the days passed and my body began to heal, I found myself reflecting on the incredible support I had received. Tee had been my rock throughout the pregnancy, staying by Lion's side while I fought for my life. I thought of the nurses, whose kindness and professionalism never wavered, even in the darkest moments. Then there were the doctors, who'd made the quick decisions that had saved me. Lastly, was the stranger, a mother I had never met, whose words had given me strength at a time when I had none left.

In those quiet moments, as I regained my strength bit by bit, I clung to hope. The road ahead was still uncertain, and the challenges were far from over, but we had made it thus far. Lion had survived his battle against

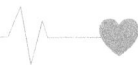

his heart condition, and I had survived mine against the haemorrhage. We had both come so close to the edge, yet there we were, still standing, still fighting.

The days stretched on, filled with moments of worry, hope, and healing. I knew there would be more surgeries, more hospital stays, more sleepless nights ahead, but I also knew that I wasn't alone in my fight. With the unwavering support of Tee, the medical staff, and the network of parents who understood our journey, I found the courage to take each day as it came.

Lion and I had fought hard to be there, and we would continue to fight, side by side, every single day. It was only the beginning of our journey, but I knew, deep in my heart, that together, we were prepared to face whatever came next. We had both survived, and we would keep pushing forward, step by step, with the strength that came from love, hope and the unbreakable bond between a mother and her child.

CHAPTER 10

Days and Nights in the Neonatal Intensive Care Unit (NICU)

Following my traumatic childbirth experience, the sun rose and set with a relentless rhythm, but for me, time seemed to stand still in the dimly lit halls of the antenatal ward. Outside, life moved forward, unaware of the turmoil swirling within me. I found myself in a parallel world where hope and fear intertwined in a delicate, painful dance. Each day, the sterile scent of antiseptic filled the air, blending with the soft, steady beep of machines. Those sounds, once foreign, became my constant companions, both a source of reassurance and a haunting reminder of the uncertainty that lingered.

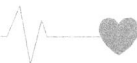

Mornings followed a familiar routine, though none of it felt routine to me. After yet another restless night spent tossing and turning in my hospital bed, I forced myself up, my heart heavy but filled with purpose. I gathered my belongings, my breast pump in hand, and prepared for the hours ahead. The pump became a symbol of my determination, of the mothering I did even when I could not hold Lion in my arms. Each session of expressing milk was bittersweet. The rhythmic hum of the machine marking my love for him, but also the distance between us. I closed my eyes and pictured his tiny face as I pumped, willing my body to nourish him, though he remained just out of reach.

That day was special, as I was finally able to see Lion after 48 long hours. My body, still weak from the ordeal, fought against me, but Tee gently wheeled me in a chair towards the NICU. Every moment felt like an eternity, but the thought of holding my baby again gave me the strength to push through. As we approached, my heart raced with both anticipation and trepidation. Stepping into the NICU felt like entering another world. Harsh fluorescent lights illuminated the room, casting a sterile glow on the maze of incubators, cots and monitors. Each baby there had their own battle, their own story of resilience. Parents sat by their sides, their faces worn with worry and exhaustion, their love for their children visible

in every glance. I realised then that we were all soldiers in the same war, fighting for our little ones with every breath, every heartbeat.

When I finally reached Lion's cot, my heart seemed to skip a beat. There he was, my tiny warrior, his chest rising and falling with each fragile breath. He was swaddled in a sea of wires and tubes, yet to me, he was perfect. As I reached through the cot's opening and placed my hand on his warm, delicate chest, a surge of emotion overtook me. Tears blurred my vision as I whispered, 'Hey, Lion, my little fighter—Mummy's here.' In that moment, everything else faded: the machines, the noise, the fear. All that mattered was the warmth of his body beneath my hand, the connection between us that no distance or medical equipment could sever.

After spending several hours by Lion's side, it was time to return to my room and continue my recovery.

As Tee wheeled me back, a new wave of anxiety washed over me at the thought of leaving Lion in the NICU being cared for by strangers, albeit highly trained healthcare professionals. The idea of leaving my baby in their hands felt foreign, even terrifying, and I couldn't shake the fear. 'How can I trust them?' I confided in Tee, my voice trembling with uncertainty.

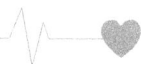

'They're experts, babe,' he reassured me, wrapping his arms around me. 'They've seen it all. They know what to do. We just have to believe in them.'

I wanted to believe him, but the fear lingered. Seeing Lion, so small and vulnerable in his little cot, made it hard to relinquish control. 'What if they don't care for him the way we would?' I whispered to Tee.

He squeezed my hand gently, his gaze steady. 'They will care for him, I promise. Trust the process. We must focus on healing so we can be there for him when he needs us.' In that moment, I realised that I had to let go of my fears and trust the professionals who had dedicated their lives to caring for babies like Lion.

I wheeled myself to the NICU every single day and night. Tee pushed me when he was around, but most of the time he was with Milo and Hugo, who had yet to meet Lion. He wanted to make sure they didn't feel our absence too much. I spent hours by Lion's side, watching his every move and listening to the soft sounds he made, savouring every moment with him.

The nurses and doctors moved with quiet efficiency, tending to Lion and the other fragile lives around him. They were incredible, taking the time to explain his care to

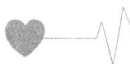

me with patience and compassion. They taught me how to change his diaper, adjust his blankets, and understand the labyrinth of monitors that tracked his every vital sign. I clung to their every word, absorbing it all as if those moments contained the most precious lessons I would ever learn. The knowledge, those acts of care; I held onto the hope that one day, when I brought him home, I would finally be the mother I always longed to be.

And so, I continued to fight alongside him. Every visit to the NICU, every drop of milk expressed, every whispered word of encouragement was my way of telling him we were in it together. Though the road ahead was uncertain, and the days stretched on in an endless blur, I knew one thing with unwavering certainty: Lion was a fighter, and so was I. Together, we would make it through this, one day, one heartbeat, one breath at a time.

The emotional toll of this experience weighed heavily on me, an unrelenting cloud that lingered through every waking moment. I was constantly on edge, battling anxiety as I waited for updates on Lion's progress. Each time a nurse walked towards me, my heart skipped a beat. Would it be good news or another challenge to overcome? My mind swirled with endless questions—was he eating enough? Were his oxygen levels stable? Was he gaining weight? As the days passed, I learnt to ride the emotional

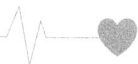

rollercoaster of NICU life, grasping onto moments of joy amidst the overwhelming uncertainty.

Nights were the hardest. As the sun set and the hospital quietened, the vulnerability intensified. The silence was suffocating, and I was left alone with my thoughts, my fears and the gnawing emptiness that filled the space where my baby should have been. I sat in my dimly lit wardroom, mechanically pumping milk for Lion, tears streaming down my face. Every drop of milk was a gesture of pure love, but it also served as a painful reminder that I was not holding him, not comforting him with my presence. The room felt hollow, reflecting the ache in my heart. I longed to feel his small, fragile body against mine, but instead, I was confined to an endless cycle of waiting and worrying.

I often stole glances at Lion through the tiny window of his cot, watching the rise and fall of his chest. In those quiet moments, I reminded myself of the strength he possessed—this tiny, fierce fighter who had already faced more battles than most. As I watched him sleep, I clung to the hope that one day, we'd be home, a family united, but the uncertainty of that future weighed heavily. What would life look like when we were finally out of the hospital? Would the fear ever leave?

One night, as I sat by Lion's side, I pulled out my phone and scrolled through pictures of our family, my other two children, and their innocent smiles shone through the screen. I longed for the day when we would all be together again as a complete family of five. I sent a quick message to Tee, letting him know how much I missed him and the kids. 'I can't wait for Lion to come home. I just want to hold him,' I typed.

His reply was almost immediate, full of love and encouragement: 'We'll get through this together. He's strong, just like his mum.'

Those words sunk deep into my heart, reigniting a spark of determination within me. I was reminded that I was not in this alone. We were a team, bound by our love for Lion and our other two children. Together, we'd fight for him, for our family, supporting each other every step of the way.

Then, a flicker of hope arrived. After a few days in the NICU, Lion was transferred to the High-Dependency Unit (HDU). It was a step-down but still full of the uncertainties of recovery. The news brought a sense of relief, though we knew there was still a long road ahead. When my brother, Finn, brought Milo and Hugo to meet their baby brother, the room was full of pure joy and love.

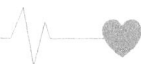

Their little faces lit up with wonder as they planted kisses on Lion's cheeks and curiously asked about the wires and tubes attached to his tiny body. For a moment, it felt like a glimpse of the future we so desperately hoped for: our family, together.

Lion was still fighting, and with every battle won, our hope grew stronger. The doctors warned us there were still many hurdles to clear: more tests, more scans, possible surgeries. Yet in those moments of sibling love and connection, I felt the weight of the struggle begin to lift.

While in the HDU, Lion underwent a series of echocardiograms and computed tomography (CT) scans, each one a test of our patience and faith. I was battling my own health issues, with blood pressure spikes that left me dizzy and drained, but even as I fought my own battles, I continued to advocate for Lion, demanding answers and pushing for his care.

Each day brought new changes, and I watched in awe as Lion fought and won battle after battle. I was finally able to hold him close, the warmth of his tiny body against mine feeling like a miracle. The first time I bottle-fed him with the expressed milk, my heart swelled with pride. 'Look at you, my little warrior,' I whispered, watching him latch onto the bottle with determination.

Just two days later, I had the incredible experience of breastfeeding him. It felt so natural, as if we were always meant to share that moment together. Yet with each joyous milestone came the dreaded reality of having to leave him to return to my wardroom.

'Mummy has to go now, but I'll be back soon, okay?' I whispered, my voice catching in my throat as I placed him gently back into his cot. Lion softly cooed as if sensing my hesitation, and I couldn't help but feel torn between my instinct to stay and my need to care for myself.

Fortunately, the HDU team made the process easier for our family. They communicated with us clearly and compassionately, explaining every step of Lion's care and progress. 'You're doing an amazing job,' one of the nurses reassured me one day. 'Every little bit helps him grow stronger.'

With all the uncertainty surrounding Lion's situation, I found solace in my university assessments. Completing and submitting my work became a way to momentarily escape hospital life. I remember sitting in my room, the soft hum of the machines outside my window, my laptop resting on my knees. 'I can do this,' I whispered to myself, focusing on the task at hand.

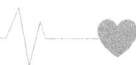

While I navigated the turbulent emotions, I learned to appreciate every small victory. I felt grateful for my family and close friends who kept in constant communication. Ava and Clara checked in on me almost every day, sending messages filled with love and encouragement. 'You've got this, Mama,' Clara texted one morning. 'Lion, Milo and Hugo are lucky to have you.'

Some family members even cooked homemade meals and brought them to the hospital for us. One afternoon, Carter, one of my relatives, arrived with a warm pepper soup. 'I thought you could use a little taste of home,' he said, his eyes bright with hope. As I savoured the meal, I felt a wave of gratitude wash over me. Those small gestures reminded me that I wasn't alone in this journey; I had a whole army of support behind me, cheering me on as I fought for my little fighter.

Then came the day I never expected. There was a multidisciplinary team (MDT) meeting, a collaborative discussion involving professionals from different specialties and disciplines who come together to plan and coordinate patient care. These meetings are common in healthcare settings, particularly in areas like oncology, paediatrics and cardiology, where complex cases require input from various experts.

Following the meeting, the cardiac consulting doctor informed me of the outcome, which left me in disbelief. After reviewing all of Lion's tests and observations, they decided that he could be discharged. No immediate intervention was needed. Lion was doing well enough to go home. I sat there, stunned, as the cardiac consultant relayed the news. I could hardly process it. After all the uncertainty, the sleepless nights and the endless fears, here was the news I had barely dared to hope for.

My brother's words from weeks earlier echoed in my mind. He had told me to keep hope alive, that Lion would be home soon. At the time, it felt like a distant dream, but now it was real. As Finn prepared to fly back home, his encouragement and faith lingered with me. Now, it was happening. I couldn't believe it. The day we longed for, the day I feared would never come, was finally here.

We had fought so hard for that moment, and now, our little fighter was proving that miracles could happen.

Nine long days after Lion's birth, the long-awaited moment finally began to take form. The hospital staff gathered around me, discussing Lion's upcoming discharge. Each update they gave filled me with a sense of hope, yet a thread of uncertainty still wove its way through my heart. I listened intently as they explained

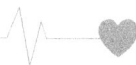

the medications, feeding schedule, signs to watch for, follow-up appointments, and the care plan we would need to establish once he was home, nodding as I tried to absorb every detail. Inside, I was a torrent of emotions: excitement mingled with fear.

I had endured so much to reach that point, and now I was finally holding my son, feeling the warmth of his tiny body against my chest without any wires between us. It was a bittersweet reminder of the journey we had travelled together, a testament to our resilience and strength. My blood pressure, which had spiralled during the worst of it, was now under control. For the first time, the future felt a little less daunting and a lot more hopeful.

Lion was discharged to me in the maternity ward while I was still an inpatient due to the complications I had following childbirth. I was monitored daily, and with each passing day, my condition continued to improve. At last, the moment I had longed for came when the nurse informed me I would be going home soon, just ten days after my world had been turned upside down. I could hardly believe it. After everything I had faced—the endless nights filled with worry and whispered prayers in the dark—the moment I'd hoped for was finally within reach. I could already envision our family together, feeling

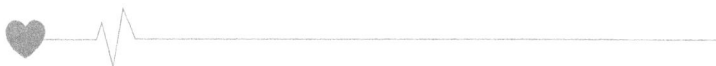

the warmth of love that had been temporarily stifled by distance and anxiety.

The preparations for my discharge felt surreal, as if I were living in a dream. The nurses helped me gather the necessary supplies, ensuring I had everything I needed for Lion's care at home. My mind spun with the flood of information, but my heart swelled with anticipation. Each detail brought me one step closer to being with my family, to feeling whole again.

As I prepared to leave the hospital, I took one last lingering look at the ward, the NICU, and the HDU room that had served as both a sanctuary and a battleground. That place had witnessed our journey, filled with tears, laughter, hope and fear. It taught me about the fragility of life and the incredible strength of love. I couldn't help but feel a pang of sadness for the parents still fighting alongside their little ones, their stories woven into the fabric of the space. Their struggles echoed in my heart, a reminder of the collective fight we all shared as parents, united in love and determination.

Finally, cradling Lion in my arms as I walked out of the hospital, my heart burst with joy and gratitude. A kaleidoscope of emotions surged within me. The weight of uncertainty still lingered, but I knew we would

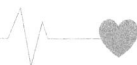

face whatever challenges lay ahead together. As I stepped outside, the sun shone brightly, casting a warm, golden glow over us. It was the beginning of a new chapter, one filled with love, hope and the promise of brighter days ahead. Lion and I were going home, and we were ready to embrace whatever life had in store for us, hand in hand, heart to heart.

CHAPTER 11

A Bumpy First Year

Being discharged from the hospital marked the beginning of a new chapter for us, yet Lion's first year unfolded like an emotional battleground, with moments of joy intertwined with constant uncertainty. Each day brought a delicate balance between hope and fear as we navigated the complexities of his health. Knowing how fragile his condition was, I became hyper-vigilant, determined to protect him at all costs. The advice we received at discharge echoed in my mind: any illness could pose a serious threat to him, especially after his time in the NICU. The heightened awareness led me to strictly limit visitors. Whenever family or friends wanted to stop by, I pointedly asked, 'Do you have a cold? A cough?' Lion was vulnerable, and the fear of his contracting an infection constantly loomed over me. The instinct to shield him

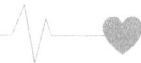

from potential harm often conflicted with my desire to share my joy with others, leaving me torn between protecting my baby and opening our doors.

I remember how coming home brought with it a rush of emotions; each one intense in its own way. I was overwhelmed with gratitude each time I held Lion close, breathing in the sweet scent of his soft skin, marvelling at the miracle of his life, but beneath the surface lurked the anxiety of the unknown. Would he stay healthy? Would we end up back in the hospital? These questions occupied my mind, but I pushed them aside, choosing instead to focus on the love that filled our home.

The first year of Lion's life was an unrelenting rollercoaster of hospital admissions and medical evaluations. Each visit brought a fresh wave of anxiety as we faced recurring chest infections and the ongoing challenges of his condition. The journey was not only a test of Lion's strength but also a profound challenge for our entire family. The early weeks were a blur of adjusting to life with a newborn while juggling the needs of my two older children. Their laughter echoed throughout our home, a comforting reminder of normalcy amidst the chaos. I cherished the small moments: late-night feedings, the gentle rise and fall of Lion's chest as he slept and the adoring kisses from his siblings.

Caring for Lion at home was a labour of love full of tender moments and constant care. Each day, I poured my heart into ensuring his comfort and well-being, cherishing every little milestone while navigating the challenges of his condition. One moment stood out vividly in my memory, capturing the weight of Lion's condition and the challenges we faced together. During his feedings, I noticed that Lion sweated profusely, his tiny body damp as he struggled through each bottle. His breathing was laboured, and every breath felt like a battle. My heart ached watching him work so hard for something that should have been effortless. He also had frequent blue episodes, particularly when he cried, where his lips and skin would take on a dusky, almost cyanotic hue. Alarmed, I immediately informed his cardiology team about these episodes, fearing the worst.

The cardiologists explained that these troubling symptoms were directly tied to his heart condition, a result of the reduced flow of oxygenated blood to his lungs. The pulmonary atresia and VSD, along with the complex web of MAPCAs, meant that Lion's heart had to work incredibly hard to circulate enough oxygenated blood throughout his body. The blue episodes while crying were caused by a temporary drop in oxygen saturation exacerbated by the physical exertion of his cries. It was

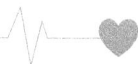

a harsh reality I had to face; every breath he took was more laborious than for most babies.

That was why he remained under the care of local community nurses, who monitored his oxygen saturation levels twice a week, ensuring they stayed within a safe range. They provided a lifeline of support, but the weight of the responsibility as his primary caregiver never left me. Every feeding, every cry, every restless night felt like a reminder of the fragility of his health. While other mothers might worry about colic or sleepless nights, my concerns were whether Lion's heart could withstand the strain of another day.

Despite these challenges, I found ways to adapt. I learnt to read his cues to understand when his little body was getting tired and needed rest. The community nurses became a crucial part of our lives, providing reassurance and helping me navigate the complexities of his care, but the hardest part was managing the constant anxiety, knowing that something as simple as a feeding or a crying spell could put an unbearable strain on his heart. Those moments turned the ordinary routines of motherhood into battles I never expected to face.

As the weeks turned into a month, cracks in our new routine began to appear. Lion developed a persistent cough, a raspy sound that sent a chill down my spine with every wheeze. Lion had always had a continuous cough since being discharged from hospital; however, this one felt different. At first, I brushed it off, telling myself it was just a cold, but deep down, I knew better. A visit to our local general practitioner reassured me that it was nothing to worry about. 'He's just building his immune system,' she said calmly, but as the cough worsened, I couldn't shake the feeling that something was wrong.

When the cough turned into wheezing, I rushed Lion to A&E, where he was admitted for four days with bronchitis. He was given antibiotics and placed on oxygen to stabilise his breathing. That hospital stay was only the beginning—Lion would be admitted many times over the months that followed for recurrent chest infections and bronchitis, living much of his first year on antibiotics.

One day, after yet another GP appointment where I was told not to worry, I still couldn't shake the unease. I contacted the community nurse, who came to check Lion's oxygen levels. When she arrived, her expression confirmed my worst fears: Lion's oxygen saturation was dangerously low. Together, we called for emergency services, and we soon found ourselves back at the hospital. The emergency room had become hauntingly familiar, with its harsh fluorescent lights, its beeping machines,

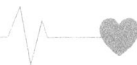

and the ever-present smell of disinfectant. I sat beside Lion, my heart heavy with worry, as the nurses worked swiftly to stabilise him.

'Mum, we've been able to stabilise Lion by giving him oxygen. Right now, we'll need to transfer him to a specialist hospital, where he'll be admitted to the Paediatric Intensive Care Unit (PICU) for observation,' the doctor said gently.

I nodded, swallowing the lump in my throat. It wasn't the first time we'd been there, and the memories flooded back: the long, sleepless nights waiting for answers, the gnawing fear of what might happen next. As Lion was transferred to the Royal Brompton Hospital, the weight of it all threatened to crush me, but I stayed by his side, holding on to hope, even when the fear felt overwhelming.

Lion was admitted, and the cycle began again, days blending into nights as we settled back into the familiar rhythm of hospital life. The sterile smell of disinfectant, the relentless beep of the machines, and the soft hum of nurses' voices became the backdrop to our existence. I found myself moving through the motions in a daze, trying to stay strong for Lion and Milo and Hugo. I set up a small corner in Lion's hospital room, decorating it with toys and books to carve out a sense of normalcy for him. It was a small comfort amidst the flurry of medical procedures, but it made the space feel more like ours, even if for just a moment.

The impact of Lion's health challenges rippled through our entire family. I saw it in the quiet questions Milo and Hugo asked, the way their laughter sometimes fell silent when they realised we weren't going home anytime soon. I knew I had to help them navigate their feelings to keep them informed in a way they could understand. It was crucial to involve them in this difficult journey to ensure they didn't feel left behind. I explained Lion's situation gently, choosing words that made sense to their young minds. I emphasised that he was receiving the best care and the doctors were helping him get better. When the day finally came for them to visit him in the PICU, I prepared them for what they would see: beeping machines, wires attached to their little brother and doctors in scrubs bustling around. I wanted to protect them from fear while showing them that their brother was in good hands.

As we walked into the room, I held their hands tightly, offering comfort through my grip. 'Lion is very brave,' I whispered, 'and we are here to support him together.' Their wide eyes took in the sight before them, and I saw a mix of curiosity and concern on their faces, yet their love for their brother shone through. Milo reached out

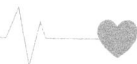

to gently touch Lion's hand while Hugo stood there quietly, watching the machines with fascination. It was a delicate balance trying to foster their connection to Lion while managing their fears, but I hoped that sharing this experience together would strengthen the bond that would hold us all through the storm.

Despite their age, Hugo and Milo sensed the shift in our family dynamic. They might not have fully grasped the gravity of what was happening, but they felt the weight of uncertainty lingering in the air. There were heartbreaking moments when they asked, 'When is Lion coming home?' or 'Why do we have to stay here so long?' Each question sliced through me, a painful reminder of the innocence they were losing all too soon. Their world had been turned upside down, and I was desperate to shield them from the worst of it, even as I navigated my own fear and exhaustion.

To keep them connected to Lion, I tried to involve them in his care whenever possible. One afternoon I asked, 'Do you want to help me make a card for Lion?' Their faces lit up with excitement, and they were soon gathered around, markers and stickers in hand, pouring their creativity into a card that would brighten their brother's hospital room.

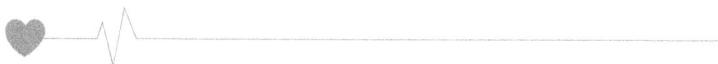

Milo always the artist, proudly held up his masterpiece. 'Look, Mummy! It's a lion!' he exclaimed, showing off a colourful lion painting on the card. I couldn't help but smile, a wave of gratitude washing over me for his ability to find joy in the smallest of things.

In those moments, love became our anchor. Even amidst the uncertainty and fear, there was still room for laughter, creativity and hope. Milo and Hugo reminded me that, despite everything, we were still a family and love could grow even in the most difficult circumstances. Watching them pour their hearts into something as simple as a card for Lion reminded me that, while I couldn't control everything happening around us, I could nurture the love that bound us together.

Those small gestures—painting a card, holding hands, whispering reassurances—became our way of fighting back against the fear. Each time we stepped into that hospital room, we carried with us the strength of a family determined to weather the storm together. Though the road ahead was uncertain, I knew that as long as we had each other, we could face whatever came next.

As the days gradually turned into weeks, it became painfully clear that this was no ordinary illness. Lion's history of frequent hospitalisations for chest infections

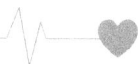

and bronchiolitis had seemed like mere preludes to something far more serious. The doctors conducted a barrage of tests and scans, each one an agonising reminder of my helplessness as I watched them poke and prod, searching for answers. Every test brought a fresh wave of uncertainty, and though I clung to hope, praying for a straightforward solution, I felt the gravity of the situation deepen with each passing hour.

Then came the day that shattered my fragile calm. I sat beside Lion, a knot of dread tightening in my stomach as I waited for yet another test result, this time, the findings from his CT scan. When the doctor finally approached, her face was a mixture of compassion and concern. 'We've found something,' she began, her voice steady yet weighted with seriousness. 'There's an artery compressing Lion's airway. It could explain the recurrent infections and breathing difficulties.'

My heart sank as her words hit me. I tried to absorb the news, but the world around me blurred. The implications were overwhelming, and the thought of my tiny baby facing yet another uphill battle felt unbearable. Tears pricked my eyes, but I forced myself to stay composed — I had to be strong for Lion.

The weeks that followed were a cascade of consultations and discussions about treatment options, leaving me feeling trapped in a waking nightmare as I struggled to regain control amidst the chaos. Each day brought new challenges, but I made sure Lion received the specialised care he needed. He was placed on high-flow oxygen to maintain safe levels, while I juggled trips back and forth between the hospital, my placement, school runs for my other children and managed Tee's unpredictable work shifts.

One day, on my way to drop Hugo at nursery, I ran into Ethan, a family friend. When he asked about Lion, university, and family, I struggled to explain. As I tried to put my feelings into words, tears welled in my eyes. Ethan noticing my distress, gave me a comforting hug before offering me a gentle smile and some much-needed encouragement: 'Take it easy. This chapter will pass one day,' he assured me. His words lifted my spirits, reminding me that even in the darkest times, there was still hope to cling to.

At the nursery, I knelt down to hug Hugo goodbye. He kissed me and darted off to join his friends, glancing back just long enough to say, 'I love you, Mummy!'

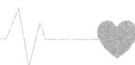

With a full heart, I replied, 'I love you, too, Hugo.' As I walked away, I inhaled deeply, grounding myself in the idea of taking each day one step at a time, holding onto hope even as I navigated this relentless storm.

As Hugo's third birthday drew near, a bittersweet ache filled my heart. The milestone, one I had hoped to celebrate with balloons, candles, and his favourite people gathered around, would have to unfold without us at home. Lion was still in the hospital, his journey far from over, and though I wanted nothing more than to be home for Hugo, I knew where I was needed most. Determined not to let the day pass without something special, we sent a cake to Hugo's nursery so he could celebrate with his friends. His teachers promised us they'd make it a joyful day, and we held onto the hope that we'd all be home together soon and celebrate as a family.

In the hospital, it was difficult to reconcile the joys of one child's birthday with the pain of watching another fight to breathe. Seeing Lion, his tiny body hooked up to machines, stirred every emotion within me. His strength amazed me, yet the endless routines of medical procedures and beeping monitors chipped away at my heart. One evening, I sat beside Lion's bed, holding his little hand, and he gazed up at me with a soft smile as if to say he knew I was there for him. It was the tiniest gesture,

but in that moment, it meant everything. I closed my eyes and let the sound of the monitors, once overwhelming, settle into a kind of melody—a rare moment of peace—reminding me that even in our darkest moments, there was something to hold onto.

During those long hospital days, the love and support from our friends and family became my backbone. Messages flooded in with words of encouragement, serving as a lifeline for my wavering resolve. My mum and my sister Chloe even flew in from abroad to be with us during that difficult time. They were often by Lion's side in the hospital, filling the room with the warmth and comfort that only family can bring. They stayed through both the quiet and challenging moments, taking turns sitting with Lion, holding his tiny hands, and singing softly to him. Their presence was a constant source of comfort, wrapping us in kindness and reminding me that we were not alone in our fight.

As the weeks unfolded, I tried to balance hospital life with my other responsibilities. Each morning brought a new flicker of hope as the medical team tirelessly adjusted Lion's treatments and medications, watched his progress and adapted their plans. Slowly, almost imperceptibly at first, Lion began to show signs of improvement. The slightest shifts—his oxygen levels stabilising or a less

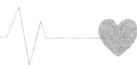

laboured breath—felt monumental. This glimmer of progress, however small, sparked something within me. It reminded me that the pain and fear weren't permanent and that maybe, just maybe, we could get through this.

As the year drew to a close, just when I had begun to accept our extended stay at the hospital, the doctor approached with news that brought me to my knees in gratitude: Lion's lungs were finally showing significant improvement. Although his airway couldn't be fully addressed yet due to his heart condition—since the artery wrapped around his airway was one of the MAPCAs supplying oxygenated blood to his lungs—he was stable enough to go home. That same artery, the doctor explained, was likely responsible for his recurring infections, leaving one of his lungs compromised. 'We can't address the airway issue until his corrective open-heart surgery,' she said, 'but for now, he's ready to go home.'

The weight of relief washed over me as I whispered, 'Thank you.' After a month of uncertainty, a month of standing watch as my child fought to breathe, we were finally going home. The reality of it felt surreal, like something I had dreamt about so often that I wasn't sure it was real when it finally happened.

After spending a month in the hospital, leaving was a bittersweet mix of joy and heartache. I glanced back at the building that had been our home and refuge, its walls bearing witness to some of our most vulnerable moments. With Lion bundled in my arms, I stepped outside into the crisp winter sunlight, bathing both of us in a warmth I hadn't felt in weeks. For the first time in what felt like forever, I could imagine a future beyond those walls.

Returning home brought its own challenges. The first few nights, I barely slept, consumed with anxiety as I lay beside Lion, listening to every cough, every tiny movement. I found myself hovering, constantly checking his breathing and watching him as if he might fade away in an instant. I knew time hadn't stopped for the rest of the world, but for me, everything felt fragile, like we were still teetering on the edge.

Despite the lingering worry, our home was full of love. Lion's siblings ran to him the moment he was home, arms open wide, showering him with hugs and giggles. Their laughter echoed through the house, filling every corner with warmth and joy, a melody that lifted my spirits and reminded me that family was a source of healing. They kissed him, babbled to him about all he'd missed. Though Lion was still recovering, his smile said it all.

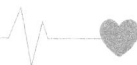

As we began to settle into our new normal, I found myself reflecting on the year we'd just survived. Lion's first year had been nothing like I had expected, each step along the way full of trials I never could have foreseen. The road was bumpy, yet it was also a journey that deepened our love and resilience. Looking at my son, I knew he was a fighter, his spirit unbroken by even the most relentless of challenges.

In that season of healing and growth, I held tightly to the belief that Lion was a warrior and that our family had grown stronger. We would take things one day at a time, cherishing each small victory and finding comfort in one another. The future might still hold uncertainties, but we were ready to face them together, drawing strength from the love that bound us. In the meantime, we would celebrate every precious moment, finding light even in the shadows and knowing that in the face of adversity, our family would always find a way to shine.

CHAPTER 12

Diagnostics Procedure

Lion's first year was a relentless test, every moment filled with the unknown, every day a reminder of both his fragility and his astonishing strength. Life was anything but typical from the second he was born. We were thrust into a world of specialised care, medical crises, and tiny but hard-fought victories that made our ordinary moments feel extraordinary. Each diagnosis, hospital admission, and update from his doctors redefined what it meant to be strong, and I quickly found that 'strong' was a word I'd need to live by if I was going to get through our journey by his side.

When Lion was just seven months old, our family was rocked by yet another hurdle. Following his one-month-long hospitalisation, a detailed scan revealed that an

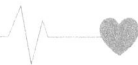

artery was pressing against his airway, which was likely the cause of his frequent chest infections. The cardiology team advised a cardiac catheterisation to get a closer look at his heart and assess whether his fragile system could withstand the next steps in his treatment. During one of our consultations, the cardiologist explained, with both compassion and precision, that this procedure would help them understand how his heart was functioning and determine whether he could undergo a full repair or if he'd need a partial fix, a decision that might mean another open-heart surgery later to close the ventricular septal defect, or VSD, in his heart.

The news hit like a tidal wave, leaving me breathless. As the doctor spoke, I found myself trying to hold back the dread that threatened to consume me. On the day of the catheterisation, I held Lion close, whispering soft reassurances as we prepared for what would be his most significant procedure yet. 'You're so brave, my little warrior,' I murmured, holding him so tightly I felt his every heartbeat, every breath. When the medical team came to wheel him into the procedure room, a piece of me went with him, and my heart felt as fragile as his tiny body. Each second in the waiting room felt like an eternity, the ticking clock a reminder of the weight we carried, the uncertainty we faced.

Finally, after hours that seemed to stretch endlessly, the doctor returned. Her expression was a mixture of reassurance and concern. 'Lion did well,' she said, her voice carrying a trace of both relief and worry. 'There are still things we need to monitor, but he's stable for now.' Relief flooded over me, but I knew it was only a temporary victory—we were still on a journey with many unknowns, each one casting a shadow over the moments of relief.

Lion was discharged the same day he had his catheterisation. It was a day filled with mixed emotions. I was both relieved and anxious, but at least we were leaving the hospital together, ready to face the next stage of our journey.

Shortly after his catheterisation, we had an appointment with the consultant to discuss the results in full detail. The doctor explained that while Lion would eventually need surgery, there was still uncertainty as to whether it would be a full repair or a partial one. He explained that the decision would depend on the surgeon on the day of the surgery, who would consider the size of the MAPCAs (major aortopulmonary collaterals) and other factors before making his final choice.

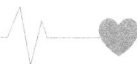

As he spoke, I tried to take it all in, but deep down, I held onto one hope: that the surgeon would perform a full repair. I clung to the belief that the strength Lion had shown on this journey would continue to help him fight his way through it. He had already proven himself to be a warrior, and I knew he wouldn't give up.

Back at home, Tee and I began to process the catheterisation results and the consultant's appointment. The weight of it all still felt heavy on my chest, but there was a sense of calm, too, a quiet hope that the future might hold something better for our little fighter. As we sat together, I couldn't help but reflect on everything we had been through. There was a long road ahead, but we were ready to face it together, with Lion leading the way.

In the week after Lion's catheterisation procedure, what began as a small, nagging cough quickly spiralled into something more serious. At first, I dismissed it as just a minor irritation, something that would pass on its own, but as the days went by, the cough worsened, and soon, his breathing became laboured. Before we knew it, Lion was hit with recurring chest infections, each one more persistent and harder to shake than the last.

It didn't take long before we were back in the hospital, and the feeling of helplessness crept in a little more as it

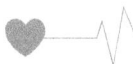

did with each returning visit. I remembered the first time we returned—Tee and I had rushed to the emergency room, both of us silently panicking, not knowing what to expect. As we waited for the doctors to take over, a sense of heaviness settled over me, though their calm faces offered little comfort.

'Do you think he's going to be okay?' I asked Tee quietly as we sat in the cold hospital room, my fingers tightly gripping his.

He didn't answer right away. His eyes were locked on Lion, who was hooked up to machines, struggling to breathe. 'I don't know,' Tee finally said, his voice barely above a whisper, 'but we have to trust the doctors. They'll do everything they can.'

I nodded, trying to hold on to that sliver of hope, but inside, I was terrified. Every cough, every wheeze from Lion felt like a punch to my chest. Each trip to the hospital felt like we were being pulled back into the storm we were so desperately trying to escape.

Over the next few days, we were back and forth between the hospital and home. Each stay at the hospital felt longer than the last. Doctors ran tests, administered antibiotics, and kept a close eye on his oxygen levels, but the infections

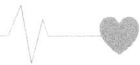

kept coming. I couldn't shake the feeling we were in a never-ending loop, trapped between hope and fear.

The constant stream of antibiotics became his lifeline, a bitter reality I had to accept. I found myself hovering by his bedside, watching his small chest rise and fall, each breath an effort, monitoring every dip in his oxygen levels, every slight change in his breathing. 'His immune system is still catching up,' the paediatrician would remind me, trying to offer some comfort amidst my growing fears.

As the infections piled up, so did the strain. The sterile halls of the hospital became a second home; the smell of antiseptic and hum of machines became as familiar as the sounds of our own home. I carried notebooks filled with medical details, each page a testament to Lion's fight, to his strength in the face of unimaginable difficulty. Each admission felt like a setback, but I forced myself to see beyond the exhaustion and worry, finding solace in even the smallest of victories: a good feeding session, a moment when his oxygen levels stabilised, a smile that made all the pain momentarily disappear.

Amidst the struggle, I found unexpected moments of pure love and joy, a fierce light in the darkness. Every time Lion's eyes met mine, there was a glimmer of resilience, an unspoken promise that we'd face this together. His

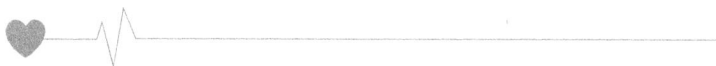

wide-eyed gaze, so full of trust, reminded me why I had to keep going. When I looked through photos of his siblings, their bright faces free of worry and full of laughter, I felt renewed. Those images became anchors, grounding me when the fear became overwhelming. Late at night, I'd send messages to Tee, trying to capture the strength I was barely holding onto. 'We're going to make it through this,' I'd type, hoping the words would be as much of a comfort to him as they were a reminder to myself.

Through it all, the support from our family and friends remained our lifeline. They continued to rally around us, their prayers, visits and messages bringing warmth to even our darkest days. Each small gesture—a thoughtful message, a moment of quiet prayer, or even a simple text to say they were 'thinking of us'—fortified my resolve. I leaned into their love and strength, feeling their support hold us up as we fought each day's battle.

Lion's first year was a journey through valleys I hadn't anticipated, yet it taught me lessons in resilience, love, and the relentless power of hope. I learned to celebrate the smallest of milestones—each time Lion's weight increased, every steady breath he took, every tentative laugh that filled the room—reminding me of the life and laughter we were fighting to reclaim. I became familiar with the blend of exhaustion and hope that defined life

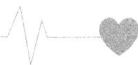

with a medically fragile child, finding joy in his courage and strength and in the love that united our family in our battle.

I often found myself reflecting on how far we had come. Lion had endured so much, yet his spirit remained unbroken, and ours grew stronger alongside his. The path ahead was still uncertain, with many challenges awaiting us, but we were ready. We had become a family bound not just by love but by resilience and a steadfast hope that we carried like a torch through the dark. Our journey was just beginning, and though I didn't know what lay ahead, I was prepared to face it, to hold on to hope and to fight for every precious moment. We had been through the fire, and together, we would face whatever came next.

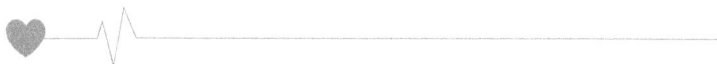

CHAPTER 13

The Unfaltering Student

Continuing my social work degree and placement amidst the chaos of life felt like trying to juggle flaming torches while riding a unicycle, a precarious balancing act that tested my limits at every turn. The relentless demands of my studies coupled with the weight of Lion's health challenges and the responsibilities of motherhood often left me breathless and overwhelmed. Yet, I was incredibly fortunate to have a solid support network in Tee, my mother, my sister Chloe and Mamita, Tee's mother. They were my steadfast support, helping me navigate our tumultuous journey with unwavering love and dedication.

Tee often returned from work tired but ready to take over without hesitation. He'd stay with the children, manage

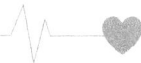

household chores and handle the shopping, giving me the precious time I needed to focus on university and my placement. I vividly remember one evening when, after a particularly exhausting day, he looked at me with determination in his eyes and said, 'You're going to graduate, and I'll be here, stepping in whenever you need.' He didn't just say it; he lived it, making sacrifices and stepping up whenever life became overwhelming. His unwavering commitment became the foundation holding our lives together, allowing me to chase my dreams even during times of chaos.

My mother was a steadfast pillar of strength during those early days, her presence a soothing balm for my anxious heart. When she arrived at my home from abroad, a wave of relief enveloped me as if the weight of the world had been lifted from my shoulders. She had an uncanny ability to sense when I was descending into despair, and she would swoop in like a superhero, ready to offer her support in whatever way I needed. Whether it was holding Lion while I caught up on schoolwork or simply being there to listen as I poured out my worries, her willingness to step in made all the difference. In moments when the weight of my responsibilities felt insurmountable, she would remind me of my resilience, gently pushing me to keep moving forward. Her encouragement was like a guiding star, illuminating the path through my darkest hours.

When my sister Chloe visited, her presence provided much-needed support. She gave me the time to focus on my studies and cherish precious moments with Lion. We also reminisced about our childhood, which helped me feel connected and uplifted during such a challenging time. Her steady support was a reminder that, even in the midst of hardship, I wasn't alone.

Mamita played an equally vital role in our lives, stepping into the maternal space with warmth and grace. From the very beginning, her love for Lion, Milo and Hugo was palpable, radiating with her every visit. She would arrive with thoughtful gifts—tiny clothes, toys and treats—just when I needed a pick-me-up. Whether preparing meals for our family or spending quality time with the kids, she entered our home like a gentle breeze, easing our burdens and reinforcing the idea that we were all in this together. She often shared stories of her own experiences, offering insights that provided me with comfort and perspective during our most challenging times. Her empathy and wisdom were like a soothing balm for my weary soul, and her unwavering presence gave me the strength to keep going.

One particularly overwhelming day stands out vividly in my memory. I was seated at the kitchen table, drowning in textbooks and notes, feeling the weight of motherhood

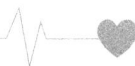

and my placement pressing on me like a heavy anchor. Just then, Mamita walked into the kitchen with a quiet, determined smile that instantly lifted my spirits. 'Go study; I've got everything here,' she insisted, her eyes sparkling with a kindness that melted my exhaustion. She began preparing dinner with practised ease, and soon, a comforting aroma filled the room.

Once dinner was ready, we settled at the table together. Her gentle presence and calm energy seemed to soothe the tension I had been carrying. Between bites, we shared stories and laughter, and as we spoke, I felt the day's stresses dissipate, replaced by a profound sense of gratitude. In those simple, quiet moments — sharing food, laughter, and connections — I found a source of hope that reminded me of life's beauty, even amidst hardship. It was these pockets of comfort that rekindled my strength, showing me that I could keep moving forward as long as I had such love and support.

Navigating the complexities of my social work placement required not only the flexibility of my supervisors but also the steadfast encouragement of my family. There were days I felt as if I was teetering on the edge of collapse, my heart heavy with the weight of conflicting demands. On those days, the unwavering belief my family held in my ability to juggle everything was a grounding force.

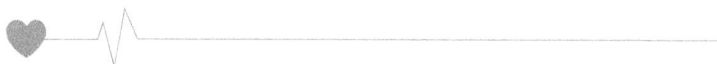

They understood my dreams and aspirations, and their support was a powerful reminder of the importance of community and connection during times of need. It was their belief in me that inspired me to reach deeper within myself, pushing past my limits to become the mother and student I aspired to be.

Through late nights spent poring over textbooks and early mornings filled with diaper changes and school runs, I found strength in knowing I was not alone. Tee, my mother, Chloe and Mamita formed an unbreakable network of support, each playing a unique role in my journey. They taught me it was not just okay to lean on others; it was essential. Asking for help became a testament to my strength, not a sign of weakness. Together, we forged a path through the chaos, illustrating that unity and support are powerful forces in overcoming adversity.

In this chapter of my life, I discovered that the path to becoming a social worker was not merely academic achievement; it was about resilience, empathy, and the relationships we built along the way. The love and support from my family and Mamita deepened my understanding of the essence of social work: advocating for others, standing strong in adversity and fostering a sense of belonging that uplifted and empowered. Each

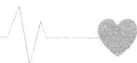

experience, each act of kindness, painted a richer picture of what it meant to care for one another.

As I moved forward in my placement, I carried their love and encouragement with me like a shield against the challenges that lay ahead. Their unwavering support continually reminded me that, no matter how difficult the journey became, we faced it side by side. I grew stronger with each challenge I faced, driven by the belief that I could navigate this chaotic world while remaining a devoted mother and an aspiring social worker. In the heart of the storm, I discovered that love and support were my greatest strengths, guiding me through the darkest nights and into the light of a new day.

CHAPTER 14

Graduation Milestone

Standing in the auditorium, cap and gown on, I felt as though I were living in a dream. After everything my family and I had endured over the past year—the sleepless nights, the terrifying uncertainty, the endless hours spent in hospitals—that day, my university graduation felt almost surreal. It was a milestone I had long worked toward, but it had never meant as much as it did in that moment. It wasn't just about earning a degree; it was about resilience, about overcoming challenges that once seemed insurmountable and about showing my children the power of perseverance.

In the months leading up to graduation, completing my degree felt nearly impossible. Lion's health was always a priority, consuming my every moment. It felt

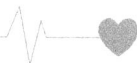

like I was surviving minute by minute, clinging to hope whilst balancing the intense demands of motherhood and academics. Between hospital visits, late-night vigils by Lion's side, and the constant anxiety of the unknown, I somehow found pockets of time to complete assignments, but each task felt like an uphill battle. There were countless times when I thought about quitting, about putting my studies on hold to focus solely on my family, yet there was a quiet, determined voice inside me that refused to give up. I wanted to show my children that no matter how dark life got, we would keep fighting, keep dreaming and keep striving.

The weeks leading up to graduation blurred together. Hospital rooms became my makeshift office, and I often reviewed my lecture notes in the dim lights besides Lion's bed. I spent my mornings on campus and my nights watching over him as he battled one infection after another. Sleepless nights became the norm, but so did my unwavering determination. Each small accomplishment felt like a triumph, whether it was submitting an assignment on time or completing a task. The more I managed to juggle, the more it felt as if I could make it work. My children needed a mother who would model strength in adversity, and I was determined to be that mother.

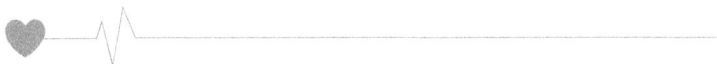

Then graduation day arrived. It seemed to come out of nowhere, just two months before Lion's scheduled open-heart surgery. It was a warm summer day in July, filled with excitement and anticipation, but I barely had time to process what the day meant, let alone prepare for it. As I stood before the mirror, adjusting my cap and gown, it felt like I was stepping into someone else's life. How could that be me? Only a short time ago, I was deep in the trenches of fear and uncertainty, unsure if I could hold everything together, yet there I was, on the verge of walking across the stage, ready to take on the moment.

This graduation wasn't just a celebration of academic achievement; it was a testament to the strength and resilience that had carried me through the darkest of times. It was proof that even in the most challenging circumstances, there was always room for hope and always a way forward. That day was for Lion, my children and the person I had become in the process. I had made it through the storm, and now I was ready for whatever came next.

As I entered the packed auditorium, I felt both excitement and anxiety build within me. My classmates were all around me, each of us bringing our own battles and triumphs into the room. We exchanged glances, our eyes reflecting an understanding of what we had all endured

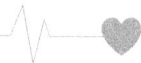

to get to that point. I spotted my family in the crowd: my father, who had travelled from afar to support me; Tee, holding a bouquet of flowers, and my children, Milo, Hugo, and Lion, were all there to witness the day.

My close friend Jill and my adopted brother Carter were there too, each holding one of my children and sharing in my joy. Seeing them by my side filled me with a deep sense of gratitude and pride. Every person in that room had been an irreplaceable part of my journey, offering support and lifting me up when I was at my lowest, helping me push forward through the toughest moments, and their presence meant more than words could express.

When my name was called, my heart raced with a mix of pride, disbelief and overwhelming emotion. Taking a deep breath, I walked across the stage, and as I did, I locked eyes with Tee. He was smiling, his face beaming with pride as he recorded the moment, mouthing, 'You did it. I'm so proud of you.' Tears welled up as I felt the significance of that shared moment. In that small exchange, I knew it wasn't just my achievement; it was ours. For every sleepless night he'd spent comforting me, for every encouragement he'd whispered when I was ready to give up, it was as much his moment as it was mine.

I smiled back at him, whispering, 'We did it.'

With my diploma in hand, I felt a wave of triumph wash over me. I had done it. Against every challenge, I had completed my degree. As I walked back to my seat, my heart soared with pride and gratitude. I thought of the countless nights I had spent studying with Lion asleep in my arms or rushing through readings during hospital visits. Every sacrifice, every ounce of determination, had been worth it. I had made it, and I felt a renewed strength inside me, knowing that whatever came next, I could face it head-on.

After the ceremony, I was enveloped by a sea of family and friends, each of them offering warm hugs, radiant smiles and words of encouragement that touched my heart. I felt their pride and love so deeply that it nearly overwhelmed me. Just then, I saw Lion toddling toward me, his little face bright with excitement. He lifted his hand and, with a slight cry, reached out, babbling, 'Mama.' Though he was young, it was as if he truly understood the depth of its meaning. I scooped him up, holding him close, his heartbeat steady and reassuring against mine, a living reminder of everything we had overcome together.

Moments later, Milo and Hugo ran over to me, their little faces beaming with pride and joy. Milo threw his arms around me, his voice ringing with admiration. 'Well done,

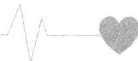

Mummy!' His words, so simple yet so heartfelt, filled me with warmth.

I bent down, wrapped my arms around Milo and Hugo and drew them close. 'Thank you, my darlings,' I whispered, my voice thick with emotion as I tried to keep the tears from spilling over. Their love, their pride — it was almost too much to contain. Those were the moments that made every struggle worthwhile, the moments that reminded me why I had persevered even when the journey felt overwhelming.

As I held all three of my children close, I felt immense gratitude for our journey and for the strength that had carried us through it. This was my family, my heart, my reason for pushing forward through every challenge. Standing there, surrounded by their love and joy, I felt as if I had truly arrived.

That evening, we gathered for a small celebration at a cosy restaurant nearby. The room was filled with warmth, laughter and love, each moment a precious memory. I looked around at the faces of my loved ones, each of them a pillar of strength that kept me going.

As we shared stories and laughter, my thoughts drifted to Lion, the little warrior who had fought so bravely against the odds. His resilience had been my greatest inspiration. My journey had become about more than just a degree — it was a mission, a promise to advocate for every family facing unimaginable challenges. I wanted to ensure that every child, every parent, had the support they needed to navigate the trials life threw their way. My graduation wasn't just a personal accomplishment — it was a symbol of hope, a beacon for families like mine who were fighting their own battles.

Later that night, as the celebration ended, I found myself reflecting on the road I had travelled to get there. Graduation wasn't just an academic achievement — it symbolised the strength of perseverance, the promise of hope, and the impact of support. Every hardship had been met with love and support; every fear had been quieted by the encouragement of those around me. I was surrounded by people who believed in me, even on the days when I struggled to believe in myself. In that moment, I knew that no matter what the future held, I had the strength and support to face it. I had come so far, and I was ready to keep going.

As I looked at Lion sleeping peacefully in my arms, I felt an immense gratitude for our journey and for the strength that carried us through it. Graduation was not just an end but the beginning of a new chapter. Armed

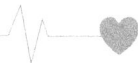

with the knowledge, skills, and unwavering support of those I loved, I was ready to step into the future with courage and hope. The road ahead would undoubtedly be filled with challenges, but I was prepared to face them, knowing that every hardship, every triumph, brought me closer to the person I was meant to be.

Surrounded by laughter and love, I made a silent promise—to Lion, Milo, Hugo, Tee and myself—that I would continue my journey with a heart full of hope and a spirit that would not break. Graduation was not just my own victory; it was a testament to the resilience of a family that had weathered every storm and emerged stronger for it. With my diploma in hand and my family by my side, I was ready to take on whatever came next, confident that together we could overcome anything.

CHAPTER 15

The Road to Surgery

As the golden days of summer slipped away after my graduation, the reality of Lion's upcoming heart surgery began to press on me more heavily. September, the month we'd marked in our minds for so long, was coming fast. The surgery, the one we'd known he would need since birth, was no longer a distant event on the horizon—it was now part of our immediate future, something that felt both inevitable and terrifying. The operation was critical. It held the key to his future quality of life. In so many ways, it was as if every fibre of my being was being pulled in two directions, both longing for it to be over and dreading what might happen.

The doctors walked me through the steps of the procedure several times. I'd researched every term, every

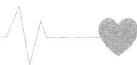

potential outcome, and clung to the success stories, but in medicine, there are no absolute guarantees, and the unpredictability gnawed at me. This wasn't just a typical surgery; it was invasive and intensive, filled with the risk of complications, each of which seemed like an insurmountable 'what if' that haunted my thoughts. What if his little heart struggled under the pressure? What if the surgery didn't go as planned? As his mother, the weight of these questions felt as vast as the ocean, and I couldn't escape the tide of fear that seemed to follow me everywhere.

The months leading up to his surgery were a strange mixture of hope and fear. Some days, I'd wake up with a sense of purpose, certain we would face this challenge and overcome it together. I told myself that I'd been through so much already: graduation, balancing motherhood with placement, navigating the storms of his first year. I was strong, and Lion was strong, too. Together, we could conquer it, but then there were days when the fear took completely over. It settled in like a fog, making it impossible to focus on anything but the looming reality of the operating room. My heart raced with anxiety, and I felt as if I were living on the edge of a cliff with no idea of what was waiting at the bottom. I wanted to protect my other children from the burden, to give them a semblance

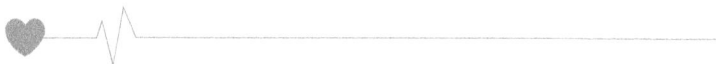

of normalcy, but that meant I had to mask my own fears, which was an exhausting feat of emotional endurance.

Despite the overwhelming anxiety, we tried to create moments of joy, and I focused on filling our days with as much love and laughter as possible. Through it all, Lion was the epitome of light and resilience. His bright eyes and playful spirit could lift the heaviest cloud. Watching him giggle at the smallest of things, seeing him babble to his siblings and witnessing his delight at the world around him gave me strength. Those joyful, seemingly ordinary moments with him were everything to me. They were small windows through which I could pretend we were just a typical family without a major surgery looming over us. In those moments, I could forget his condition, let go of my fears, and live in the present. I soaked up his smile, letting it wash over me like sunlight, and I knew then that no matter what was coming, those moments of happiness and love were the foundation that would hold us steady.

As September drew nearer, my mind was a whirlwind of emotions. I reminded myself that I'd faced challenges before and that even though this was different, I would not face it alone. My family, friends, and community surrounded me with support, and I clung to their encouragement. I had prepared as best as I could, but

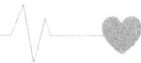

there was still an undeniable sense of stepping into the unknown.

The day before the surgery, we found ourselves shuttling back and forth to the hospital for Lion's pre-surgery assessments. Each visit felt like a countdown, a sombre reminder of what lay ahead. Every time I walked through those hospital doors, a wave of anxiety rolled over me, settling in my stomach. The doctors and nurses were incredibly compassionate, patient, and attentive as they explained each step of the procedure, yet no amount of reassurance could shake the underlying dread I felt. The surgery was the defining moment that could give my son a new lease on life, but it was also riddled with risks that haunted my every thought.

I was fixated on preparing for the hospital stay. I spent hours meticulously packing and repacking the hospital bag, running through checklists of essentials, backup plans, people to call, and arrangements for my older children. It was like gearing up for a battle, and in a sense, it was. It was the biggest fight Lion would face, and I wanted everything in order as if it might somehow keep us safe from what lay ahead.

The night before surgery, I barely slept. My mind played back all the moments leading up to that point: the

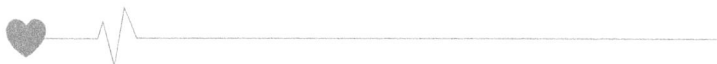

20-week scan when we first heard something was wrong with Lion's heart, the countless trips to specialists, the exhausting hospital admissions due to chest infections, and now, the monumental surgery that promised to change everything. The weight of it all felt crushing, yet in the quiet of the night, I realised how far we'd come, even though we still had a daunting journey ahead.

The hospital, had graciously offered us accommodation, knowing it would be a difficult journey to make each day from home. My dad had decided to stay with us after my graduation, lending his quiet strength and unwavering support during the days leading up to Lion's surgery. That morning, as we drove together to the hospital, the familiar roads felt profoundly different. Each passing mile brought us closer to the moment we had both dreaded and anticipated, a moment we knew was necessary but wished we could somehow avoid.

Once we arrived, we dropped my dad, Milo and Hugo at the hospital accommodation, a temporary home base for our family, while Tee and I stayed close to Lion in the hospital. As we prepared to part, my dad placed a steady hand on my shoulder, grounding me in a way only he could. Then, he knelt beside Lion and spoke to him in a low, calming tone, almost as if Lion could understand every word. 'You are strong, my boy,' he whispered, 'and

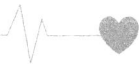

you will come out victorious.' His words lingered in the air, filling me with a deep sense of faith.

He then turned to me, his gaze unwavering, and offered a heartfelt prayer for protection and strength. It was one of those rare moments of understanding, a silent exchange that felt as though his strength had become mine.

After saying our goodbyes, Tee and I walked into the hospital, the corridors eerily quiet yet alive with the significance of the day. It struck me then, the delicate balance we were treading. On the one hand, we were praying for a life-changing surgery, one that could give Lion the future he deserved, but on the other, I couldn't shake the gnawing fear that this might be the most challenging journey we'd ever face.

Once inside, we spent the hours before surgery with Lion, trying to keep things as calm and comforting as possible. We were in his room, surrounded by the familiar beeping of monitors, with Lion's toys scattered around and an overwhelming stillness that mirrored our anxious thoughts.

The anticipation hung thick in the air, heavy with both hope and dread. The surgeon entered, exuding a quiet confidence that both comforted and unnerved me. With

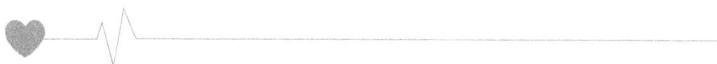

a reassuring smile, he began to explain the intricacies of the procedure once more: 'Today, we'll be performing an RV-PA conduit, which stands for right ventricle to the pulmonary artery,' he said, his voice steady and clear.

I felt a pang of urgency wash over me. The words had become familiar, yet in that moment, they bore the weight of Lion's future. 'So, what, exactly, does that mean for him?' I asked, trying to keep my voice steady as my heart raced.

The surgeon met my gaze, his expression earnest. 'Lion's condition is unique and complex. He has pulmonary atresia with a ventricular septal defect (VSD) and MAPCAs. These MAPCAs have formed to compensate for the underdeveloped pulmonary arteries that should have been there since birth. Our goal is ambitious: to create a surgical graft or tube that forms a direct pathway from his right ventricle to the pulmonary artery.'

'Will that fix the problem?' I pressed, desperate for clarity.

'Essentially, yes,' he replied. 'This procedure is often necessary for congenital heart defects, where the natural pathway between the heart and lungs is either underdeveloped, blocked or completely absent. By performing this conduit, we can improve the blood flow

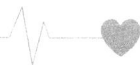

to Lion's lungs.' He paused for a moment and asked if we were following. 'Additionally, we will attempt unifocalisation, where we'll connect as many of the reusable MAPCAs as possible to create a functioning pulmonary artery system.'

'Reusable MAPCAs?' I echoed, still grappling with the complexity of it all.

'Correct. We'll only use those that are robust enough to withstand the integration,' he explained, his hands gesturing as if he were weaving the arteries together right before my eyes. 'Some MAPCAs may be too small, too fragile, or misaligned, making them unsuitable for the pathway. By uniting the viable arteries, we hope to enable Lion's heart to deliver oxygen-rich blood more effectively, improving his oxygen levels and stabilising his circulation.'

I nodded, but the seriousness of the situation hung over me. What about the hole in his heart?' I asked, my heart racing with a blend of dread and anticipation.

The surgeon's expression softened slightly. 'If feasible, I will also attempt to close the VSD, but that decision will ultimately depend on the sizes of the arteries I find once we begin the surgery.'

Taking a deep breath, I struggled to absorb all the information. 'So, it's really a matter of assessing the situation in real-time?' I clarified, hoping to grasp the enormity of what lay ahead.

'Exactly,' he replied, his eyes steady. 'I'll be examining Lion's anatomy carefully to determine the best course of action. This surgery is his best chance for a normal life, a future free from the constant struggle to breathe and the limitations that come with it.'

I felt my breath hitch at the thought of my son lying on the table, vulnerable yet incredibly strong. The image of his tiny heart exposed sent a shiver down my spine. 'Thank you,' I managed to say, my voice thick with emotion, 'for everything you're doing for him.'

'Thank you for trusting us,' the surgeon said, his tone earnest. 'We'll do everything we can to give Lion the life he deserves.'

As he finished explaining, I nodded, the magnitude of the surgery pressing heavily upon me. I took one last deep breath, clutching to the hope that day would be the turning point in Lion's journey, the catalyst for a better future.

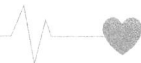

The emotions engulfed me like a storm: an overwhelming mix of pride in my son's resilience, fear of the unknown, and an unyielding hope that the surgery might finally bring him some peace. Each heartbeat felt amplified, reverberating through me as I stood there, a parent on the precipice of uncertainty. I fought to steady myself, but the intensity of it all was almost suffocating.

Taking a deep breath, I summoned the courage to voice the question that had been gnawing at me since we arrived. It was a question I was almost too afraid to ask, yet I knew I had to. 'How long will it take?' I whispered, bracing myself for the answer, my heart racing.

The surgeon met my gaze, his eyes reflecting a mixture of empathy and professionalism. 'The surgery could last anywhere from a few hours to an entire day, depending on how smoothly everything goes,' he replied, his tone steady and reassuring.

The significances of his words settled in the room, making the air feel even heavier as if the walls were collectively bracing for the long hours ahead. I felt the clock ticking away precious moments, each second pulling me deeper into the unknown.

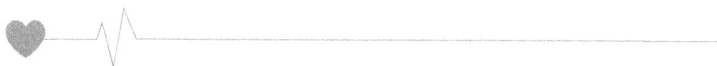

I swallowed hard, trying to wrap my mind around the time frame. 'Okay,' I managed to say, my voice barely above a whisper. I reached for the stack of paperwork outlining the risks and details of the surgery, my hands slightly trembling as I picked it up.

With a shaky hand, I signed my name, each stroke of the pen feeling like an act of both courage and surrender. As I wrote, the surgeon's earlier words about potential complications echoed in my mind, threatening to drown me in worry, but I pushed those thoughts aside, focusing instead on the path we had chosen for Lion, one filled with love, hope, and unwavering trust.

The surgeon watched me as I completed the paperwork, and when I looked up, he gave me a small, reassuring nod. It was a silent promise that they would do everything possible for my son. 'We're going to take great care of him,' he said, his voice firm yet soothing.

In that moment, I clung to his words like a beacon of hope. 'Thank you,' I whispered, my voice thick with emotion. It was a simple expression of gratitude, but it held the weight of my entire heart.

As the surgeon turned to finalise the preparations, I took a deep breath, trying to steady the whirlwind of

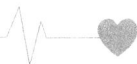

feelings inside me. I was filled with fierce determination, an unwavering belief that that day would be a turning point for Lion. Whatever lay ahead, I knew we were in it together, and for the first time that day, I allowed a glimmer of hope to break through the fear.

After he left, I held Lion close, taking in his innocent little face. He looked up at me, unaware of what was coming, with a glint of curiosity and wonder. I felt a lump rise in my throat—how could such a tiny, vulnerable person be heading into something so immense? I wanted to keep him in my arms, away from the sterile, intimidating world of the surgery, but I knew I had to let him go. I tried to focus on the hope that that was our turning point, that the surgery would give him a future free from the constraints of his heart condition. I tried to cling to that hope, but the what-ifs lingered in the corners of my mind.

The hours leading up to the operation were some of the hardest of my life. Each second seemed to drag on as we waited, surrounded by the white walls of the hospital room. We distracted ourselves by singing, playing games and reading stories, trying to create a sense of normalcy. Every time Lion giggled or smiled, it filled me with both relief and sorrow. I wanted to freeze those moments, to somehow capture his happiness and innocence and keep it untouched by the fear looming over us.

Shortly after the anaesthetist arrived, a calm and reassuring presence, she sat beside us to explain the steps ahead. She walked us through the entire process, detailing how she would carefully administer the anaesthesia to keep Lion asleep and entirely pain-free during the surgery. Her voice was steady, and as she spoke, she emphasised the meticulous monitoring of his vital signs throughout the procedure. Every heartbeat, breath and pressure level would be closely observed, ensuring his safety moment by moment.

She did not shy away from discussing the potential risks involved, addressing each with the care and clarity we so desperately needed. She explained that while the team would do everything to minimise any complications, some risks, however small, were an inherent part of such a complex operation. Hearing it all laid out was overwhelming, yet her compassion somehow made it easier to bear. She placed the consent form in front of us, explaining that signing it was our acknowledgement of the risks and putting our trust in their hands. Tee and I exchanged a long, silent look, feeling the enormity of our decision settle over us.

We took a deep breath and signed, entrusting our son to the care of the surgical team, feeling a mixture of fear, hope and determination for what lay ahead. The

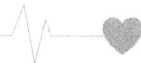

anaesthetist offered a final, comforting nod as she tucked the paperwork away, letting us know they were ready to begin whenever we were.

Finally, the moment arrived. The anaesthetist and nurses entered the room, signalling it was time to take Lion to the operating theatre. Tee and I stayed by his side as long as possible, holding his little hands and speaking softly to him. The anaesthetist team gently reassured us, explaining each step as they began to put him to sleep. My heart ached as I watched Lion's eyes close, his tiny body finally surrendering to the sedation.

Then came the hardest part: I leant down, pressed a soft kiss to his forehead and whispered, 'You've got this, Lion, my little fighter,' I murmured, my voice cracking. I felt a surge of dread as I handed him over, taking one last look at him before they wheeled him away. I watched helplessly as the doors closed between us, severing that fragile connection. The sight of him disappearing down that cold, sterile corridor broke something inside me.

The intensity of my emotions crashed down, and I couldn't hold back the tears that had been welling up inside. Tee wrapped his arms around me, his own eyes brimming with unshed tears, and gently dried my face. 'He's going to be okay,' he whispered, his voice was steady as he spoke,

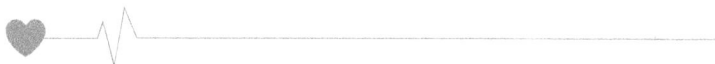

reassuring me with each word, 'Our Lion is a fighter. He will come out even stronger than before.' We clung to each other, both feeling the agonising pull of uncertainty yet drawing strength from each other's presence.

As we made our way to the waiting room, I reached for Lion's little blanket in the pram. It smelt faintly of him, and I buried my face in it, finding a small measure of comfort in its softness. We sat there surrounded by other anxious parents, but in those moments, it felt as if we were in our own world, a world where all we could do was hope, wait, and pray for our boy's safe return.

The wait felt unrelenting, each hour dragging as we tried to occupy our minds. We walked up and down the hospital corridors, our phones nearby, waiting for any update. My mind was a wildfire of thoughts, crackling with every conversation with the doctors, every smile Lion had given us, every milestone he'd reached. I thought about his first steps, his laughter, his boundless curiosity, and I held onto the hope that he would get through this, that we would get to see him grow, explore, and discover the world.

As the hours passed, I found myself looking around at the other families waiting, some visibly anxious, others quietly resolute. We were all in a strange, shared world of

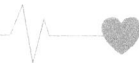

waiting, where time felt suspended, yet every second was filled with both expectation and apprehension.

As I sat in the waiting room, the minutes feeling like hours, I felt the urge to connect with, Milo and Hugo. They were just a video call away, and I needed to hear their voices, to feel that familial warmth amid the chaos. I dialled my dad on video call.

When his familiar face filled the screen, a wave of relief washed over me. 'Hey, Dad, how are Milo and Hugo doing?' I asked, trying to keep my voice steady.

'They're all doing fine,' Dad replied with a reassuring smile. 'Milo is being his usual thoughtful self."

In the background, Milo said, 'Mummy, don't worry! We're playing on our iPads, and we'll take care of each other.'

At that moment, I could almost picture Milo his eyes sparkling with determination. 'Just take care of Lion, and see you all soon,' Dad continued. I felt a surge of pride in my heart.

As if on cue, Milo leaned into the frame, his face lighting up with excitement. 'I love you, Mummy,' he exclaimed.

Hugo popped up beside him, beaming with energy. 'And I love you both more,' he chimed in, his enthusiasm infectious.

'We love you, too!' Tee and I responded in unison, laughter spilling into the call, momentarily lifting the heaviness in my heart.

'Thank you so much, Dad,' I said, gratitude flooding through me as I watched Milo and Hugo comfort each other from afar. Just seeing them safe and happy gave me a moment of solace.

Before I knew it, Milo offered a cheeky smile and waved. 'Okay, Mummy! We'll see you soon!' With that, he pressed the button to end the call, leaving me with a renewed sense of strength.

As I sat there, the warmth of their words wrapped around me like a comforting blanket. I knew that no matter how daunting the road ahead felt, the love of my family would carry me through. In that moment of connection, I found a flicker of hope, one I could hold on to as I prepared for the long day ahead.

Tee and I sat in the sterile waiting room, the ticking clock amplifying the tension hanging between us. To distract

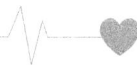

ourselves, we busied our hands with our phones, replying to a flood of supportive messages from family and friends. Each notification reminded us that we were supported by those who cared and didn't have to face this fight alone.

Ava's voice note came through, a soothing prayer for Lion that filled the space around us. I pressed play, the sound of her warm voice wrapping around us like a gentle embrace: 'Dear God, please watch over our little warrior, Lion. Give him strength and guide the surgeon's hands,' she intoned, her sincerity palpable.

As we listened, a sense of peace settled over us, easing the burden on our hearts, if only for a moment. 'Thank you, Ava,' I whispered, my heart swelling with gratitude. The combination of her prayer and our thoughts of hope created a flicker of light in the darkness surrounding us.

The hours crept by each tick of the clock echoing louder than the last. After what felt like an eternity—around 11 hours—my phone rang, and the surgeon's name flashed across the screen. A shiver ran down my spine. This was it—this was the call we had been waiting for.

'Hello?' I answered, my voice trembling slightly.

'Hi, it's Dr London,' he began. I heard the relief in his tone. 'The surgery is done, and it was successful.'

The words sent a rush of emotions flooding through me, a whirlwind of relief and gratitude mixed with an undercurrent of anxiety. 'What about the artery compressing his airway?' I managed to ask, my voice barely above a whisper, concern threading through my words.

The surgeon's response was calm and measured, providing a glimmer of hope. 'I was able to unravel it and move it away from his airway,' he said.

A wave of appreciation washed over me, and I couldn't help but exhale a breath I didn't realise I was holding. 'Thank goodness,' I exclaimed, tears of relief prickling at the corners of my eyes. 'I can't express how much that means to us.'

'We encountered a little bleeding towards the end,' he explained, 'which is why we had to stay a bit longer to stop it before leaving the theatre.'

'And Lion?' I held my breath, desperate to hear more. 'Were you able to do the full repair?'

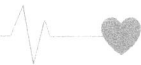

'I was able to complete the full repair,' he replied, his voice reassuring. 'The RV-PA conduit unifocalisation, and we closed the hole in his heart.'

Hearing those words ignited a wave of joy within me, and I let out a triumphant scream, tears of relief streaming down my cheeks. 'Thank you so much.' I exclaimed, overwhelmed by emotion.

'The next 48 hours will be delicate and the hardest part,' he cautioned. 'If he makes it through those hours, I believe he will be all right.'

In that moment, I felt the energy shift. 'Yes! He will be all right. He's our little fighter,' I declared, conviction swelling in my chest.

Tee and I embraced tightly, the moment heavy with gratitude and excitement. 'He made it, babe! He made it!' we said in unison, our voices tinged with joy. 'Thank God!'

The surgeon informed us that the team would let us see Lion as soon as possible and advised us to head to the PICU waiting area. We nodded, still lost in our own world of relief and happiness.

'Thank you for your dedication and care,' I replied, my heart filled with gratitude. 'You've done more than we could have hoped for.'

'Let's go see our boy,' Tee said, his eyes shining with determination.

We hurried to the PICU waiting room, our hearts racing with anticipation. We were finally on the cusp of reuniting with our little warrior, ready to support him through the next crucial steps of his journey.

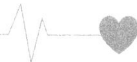

CHAPTER 16

The Aftermath of Surgery

As Tee and I sat anxiously in the PICU waiting area, the sterile hospital walls seemed to close in around us. The tension in the air was palpable. Each passing moment felt like a lifetime. We sat in silence, only able to hope and wait. Our thoughts were entirely consumed by Lion as we anxiously awaited the moment we would be called in to see him after his open-heart surgery.

Then, just as my mind spiralled with worry, the door opened, and the surgeon stepped in. Still in his scrubs, he looked slightly weary, the kind of tiredness that came with deep focus and responsibility. Following the telephone conversation, he had come to speak with us

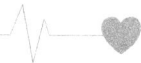

in person before heading home, a small but incredibly meaningful gesture.

He cleared his throat and began. His voice was soothing. 'As I mentioned on the phone earlier, the surgery went well.'

I barely had a second to process his words before he continued. 'The next 48 hours are crucial. Lion is at high risk for infection and other complications due to the nature of the procedure, but for now, everything is looking as it should. Keep hopeful.'

Tee and I exchanged a look of immense relief and gratitude. The impact of his words sank in, reminding us that while the surgery was behind us, the journey was far from over.

'Thank you,' I managed to say, my voice almost breaking under the strain of it all. 'Thank you for everything you've done.'

He gave a small, reassuring nod. A flicker of warmth broke through his exhausted demeanour. 'Stay strong, both of you,' he said quietly before leaving us alone with our thoughts.

It was nearly an hour later when a nurse from the PICU called us back to see Lion. My heart raced as we walked through the winding hallways and into the stark room where our son lay. Nothing could have truly prepared us for that moment. My little boy, my brave Lion, lay still on the hospital cot, his face swollen from the surgery, his small chest adorned with a clear dressing that revealed faint streaks of blood underneath. Wires, tubes and machines surrounded him, each carrying out a vital task to keep him alive.

As I took in the sight of him, a wave of emotions crashed over me: fear, relief and an overwhelming desire to comfort him. I reached out and gently took his tiny hand, feeling its warmth, though he remained still, unresponsive.

Noticing my reaction, the nurse nearby offered a gentle explanation. 'He's heavily sedated,' she said with a calm that only years of experience could bring. 'We need to keep him like this to allow his heart and body to rest fully after the surgery. He'll stay this way for around 48 hours.'

I nodded. Her words grounded me a bit, but the sight of him was still so overwhelming. Every tube and wire felt like a reminder of how fragile the moment was, yet also of the strength he carried within him. Each beep from the

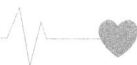

machines became a small comfort, a reminder that he was still there, still fighting.

I leaned over him, brushed my lips against his forehead and whispered, 'Lion, I'm right here. Mummy's here. I'll be with you every step of the way.' My voice quivered as I continued, 'You're so strong, my love… my little warrior.'

Tee stood beside me, his hand resting gently on Lion's tiny fingers. He whispered softly, 'You're doing amazing, son. Keep fighting. We're right here, every step.'

Together, we sat beside him, prayed quietly, and poured every ounce of our strength and love into that little room. In that moment, hope bound our hearts, fuelling us with gratitude for the medical team that had given him a fighting chance. Although the sight was hard to bear, both of us felt a burden lift. The surgery was behind us, and now we had to hold on, wait and watch over him.

After a few hours of sitting by Lion's side, absorbing each small breath, each flicker on the monitors, we finally left the PICU to reunite with my dad and our other boys. It felt as if we hadn't seen them in days, though it had only been since early that morning.

As we made our way out of the hospital, my hands instinctively reached for my phone. I began calling Ava and a few others who'd been anxiously waiting for updates.

'Ava,' I said, my voice slightly breaking as I tried to contain the wave of emotions. 'The surgery went well. Lion is in recovery now. Please, keep him in your thoughts as we get through these next days.'

A deep sigh of relief echoed on the other end of the line. 'We will,' she promised, her voice filled with warmth. 'All of us are here for you and praying for him.'

One by one, I responded to the messages that had been flooding in throughout the day. Each response felt like a release, allowing me to share the relief we felt yet keeping us grounded in the reality of what still lay ahead.

With every update, I felt our support circle wrapping closer around us, bolstering our spirits and reminding us of the journey we were on, not alone but surrounded by love, prayers and an endless well of hope.

As Tee and I began our short walk back to our family accommodation—a charity-run lodging for families with children admitted to the hospital conveniently located just

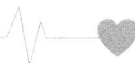

a brief stroll from the Hospital—I felt the weight of the day's events slowly pressing down on me. The building provided a temporary refuge for us, a place to regroup while our son was in the hospital. Tee reached over and took my hand, holding it firmly. In that shared silence, his hand enveloping mine, I felt the complex blend of strength and vulnerability that defined our bond at that moment. We were both deeply grateful for the medical team that had worked tirelessly to save Lion's life, yet an undercurrent of anxiety rippled through me at the thought of leaving him in someone else's care, even in the most capable hands.

'He's strong, you know,' Tee said quietly, breaking the stillness between us. 'This is just the beginning of his journey. He's in good hands.'

I squeezed his hand back and nodded in agreement, though the ache in my heart lingered. Deep down, I understood that Tee's words were meant to reassure me, but the thought of leaving Lion—despite the nurse's watchful eyes—felt like leaving a piece of my soul behind.

As we approached the accommodation, the comforting sight of the familiar building came into view, but I still felt a tug of dread. It was strange to think of returning to a space meant for rest and recuperation when my heart was still tethered to the PICU, to Lion.

When we finally reunited with Milo and Hugo, they bolted toward us, their little faces lighting up with a flurry of questions all at once. 'How's Lion, Mum?' Milo asked, his wide, earnest eyes filled with concern. 'Why didn't you bring him back with you?'

I knelt to their level, wrapped my arms around them and pulled them close. 'The doctors and nurses are taking care of him while he recovers,' I explained, trying to soften the blow of the separation. 'We'll be there every day to see him, and soon, when he's stronger, we'll all be together again.'

Milo and Hugo exchanged glances, their expressions a mix of relief and worry. I stroked their hair, feeling the heaviness of their unspoken fears pressing on my heart. They were just children, yet they seemed to carry the burden of concern far beyond their years.

'We'll have a big day tomorrow,' I continued softly, wanting to redirect their thoughts. 'You're both starting at the hospital School. It'll be a great way for you to keep learning while we're here together. For now, though, let's all try to rest, okay?'

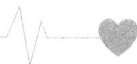

Milo and Hugo leant in, hugging us tightly before reluctantly letting go, their little bodies still radiating warmth and innocence. After they tucked themselves into bed, the quiet of the room wrapped around us. As they drifted off to sleep, I turned to my dad, who had been anxiously waiting for an update.

His wise, tired eyes searched mine for reassurance. 'How did it go, Ezy?' he asked, his voice thick with concern. I heard the tension woven into his words. As I filled him in on the surgery's outcome and Lion's recovery process, he nodded, though I could sense he was as restless as I was.

Eventually, my dad succumbed to sleep, his breathing deep, while I lay wide awake, unable to shake the unease that clung to me like a heavy fog. The reality that the surgery was over hadn't quite sunken in. Lying there in the darkness, I felt my mind circling back to the PICU and to Lion. Every nerve in my body was on edge, acutely aware that the next 48 hours would be critical for his recovery.

Unable to quell my anxiety, I began calling the nurse hourly, needing to hear of his progress, desperate for reassurance that he was still okay. Probably sensing my anxiety, one of the nurses, spoke softly to me, trying to provide comfort. 'Go get some rest,' she urged gently.

'Lion is doing just fine, and we'll update you if anything changes, I promise.'

Her words washed over me like a soothing balm, settling my frazzled nerves and easing some of my worry. With a final, grateful nod, I put down the phone and finally managed to close my eyes, allowing the exhaustion to pull me into a fragile sleep, hoping that tomorrow would bring more good news.

The next morning dawned with a sense of purpose. After a quick breakfast that felt more like an afterthought than a meal, Tee and I took Milo and Hugo to register them at the hospital School. We wanted to create a semblance of normalcy for them in this strange, uncertain environment that had become our new reality. My dad stayed back at the accommodation—only Tee and I would be visiting Lion that day. We knew we had to be cautious due to his vulnerability. Every moment felt precious, and we needed to keep our focus on Lion's recovery.

As we walked towards the school, Milo and Hugo chattered excitedly, their youthful energy a stark contrast to the unease that hung over us. I glanced at Tee, who gave me a reassuring nod, and together, we exchanged a silent vow to make that day as bright as possible for the boys.

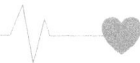

Once we'd dropped them off, Tee and I made our way back to the PICU. The air was thick with the scent of antiseptic, and the rhythmic beeping of monitors filled my ears as we entered Lion's room. The sterile environment, once daunting, had morphed into a strange sanctuary where we could be with our son, even in the quiet of our shared silence. We settled into our familiar routine, watching him, talking to him softly and offering silent prayers filled with hope for his recovery.

The PICU, with its devoted staff and constant flurry of activity, had become an integral part of our daily life. The doctors and nurses, though serious in their work, had become our allies in this journey. Each day unfolded with a similar rhythm: we visited the boys, had lunch together, and then returned to Lion's side. It was a routine that provided some structure amidst the chaos, an anchor to hold on to as we waited for Lion to grow stronger and come home.

The 48-hour mark after Lion's surgery approached, the days blended into one another, each second stretching and collapsing, blurring my sense of reality. Lion was being closely monitored. His condition required regular blood tests, X-rays and endless scans. I watched every beeping machine with a mixture of intensity and dread, clinging to the hope that each hour would bring him closer to breathing on his own.

The third day passed, and Lion remained on the ventilator, heavily sedated. The absence of progress felt like a stone lodged in my chest, and I felt Tee's unease mirroring my own.

On the fourth day, as I sat by Lion's bedside, a team of doctors approached me. The sight of their serious expressions made my stomach drop, dread pooling inside me like lead. Instinctively, I reached for my phone and called Tee, who was at the park with Milo and Hugo, along with my dad. 'Please come now,' I whispered, the tremor in my voice betraying my attempt to remain calm.

Tee rushed into the room within minutes, concern etched across his features. He took my hand and glanced anxiously at the doctors. 'What's happening?' he asked, his voice tight with worry.

One doctor stepped forward, his expression kind yet serious. 'Hello, Mum and Dad. We wanted to discuss Lion's condition and explain why he's still on the ventilator and under heavy sedation.'

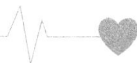

I swallowed hard, my mouth dry, my heart racing. 'Please, just tell us,' I managed, my voice barely a whisper.

The doctor nodded solemnly. 'Lion's surgery corrected many of the structural issues in his heart. However, as you know from his previous admission, we discovered that one of Lion's arteries had been wrapped tightly around his left main bronchus, which is his breathing airway. We repositioned it during surgery but,' he hesitated, choosing his next words carefully, 'that artery had been constricted around his airway for a long time. As a result, his left lung has significantly collapsed.'

My heart clenched as his words sank in. 'I thought the surgery fixed everything,' I whispered, my voice trembling. 'Isn't he okay now?'

The doctor looked at us with a gentle yet grave expression. 'The surgery corrected a lot, yes, but because that artery was pressing down on his left main bronchus for so long, it has severely compromised his ability to breathe. Right now, Lion can't breathe on his own because the left side of his airway isn't allowing enough air through.'

I felt the world spin around me. Tee squeezed my hand, anchoring me, but I could feel his fingers trembling in response to the news. He held onto me just as tightly as I clung to him.

'What... what happens next?' I managed to ask, my throat tight with fear.

The doctor's gaze softened. 'We'll need to perform more tests, including a bronchoscopy. This medical procedure allows us to view the inside of the lungs and airways. A bronchoscopy involves inserting a thin, flexible tube called a bronchoscope, equipped with a light and camera, through the nose or mouth and guiding it down into the lungs. During this procedure, we can examine the airways for any blockages, infections or other abnormalities. We may also take tissue samples, remove blockages or clear mucus. It's commonly used for diagnosing lung conditions and can be performed under local or general anaesthesia, depending on the case. This will help us see the condition of Lion's lung and left bronchus more clearly so we can plan moving forward.'

I stared at the doctor, my mind racing. 'But with all the tests he's already been through, haven't you seen anything? Can't you tell us something now?' I pleaded, desperation lacing my voice.

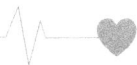

The doctor sighed. Sympathy etched across his face. 'I understand how difficult this is for you, but until we have enough information from the bronchoscopy, we can't make a definitive plan.'

I turned to Tee in utter disbelief, tears welling in my eyes. 'Babe, what is going on?' I whispered, feeling the ground shift beneath me.

The doctor asked if we had any questions before he left.

'When will you perform the procedure?' I asked, my heart racing.

'Tomorrow,' he replied, his voice filled with an undercurrent of concern.

The gravity of the situation settled around us, I held onto Tee's hand, searching for strength in his familiar warmth, hoping that the next day would bring answers and a path forward for our precious Lion.

The doctors exited the room, Tee and I turned our attention back to Lion; our hearts laden with worry. We each took one of his tiny hands and cradled it gently in our palms as we whispered words of love and encouragement. Tears blurred my vision, but I kept rubbing his hand,

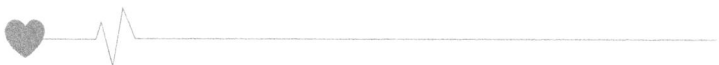

willing him to feel our presence. Then, in that poignant moment, I felt a small movement—his toes flexed ever so slightly. It was a flicker of life, a subtle reminder that he was still fighting. That tiny movement ignited a fragile hope within me, alleviating the burden of despair, if only for a moment.

After a long day, we returned to the accommodation, and Milo and Hugo, came running up to us with pure, unfiltered joy. Their little faces lit up like the sun breaking through the clouds, and as they flung their arms around us, their voices overflowing with questions.

'When can we see Lion?' Milo asked, his wide eyes shimmering with innocent curiosity.

I knelt down to hug him tightly, forcing a smile despite the heaviness in my heart. 'Soon, my love,' I said, trying to project reassurance. 'Lion is very brave, and he's working hard to get better.'

The following day blurred into a whirlwind of consultations, tests and scans, each moment feeling like an eternity. When it was time for the bronchoscopy, the airway specialist and anaesthetist approached us and handed over a mountain of paperwork detailing the risks involved. My hands slightly trembled as I leafed through

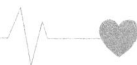

the forms, each page filled with technical jargon that only deepened my sense of dread.

Tee and I exchanged a look, our silent understanding palpable. We both knew this was a necessary step, even as signing those forms felt like we were surrendering a piece of our hearts. We signed with a collective breath, hoping it would lead us towards a clearer path for our son.

Watching Lion lay there so sedated was utterly heartbreaking. He stirred every time the medication began to wear off, as if instinctively trying to wake up. Each time, he began to rouse, panic set in, and he struggled against the breathing tube. The nurses rushed in to increase his sedation, and he slipped back into a deep, restless sleep. It was agonising to witness our little boy caught between survival and suffering, his tiny body fighting against the very thing that was keeping him alive.

Finally, the time came for the bronchoscopy procedure. The procedure which was over relatively quickly, but the waiting felt like an eternity. Tee and I sat together, our hearts heavy with dread, holding hands and praying silently.

When the doctors finally approached to speak with us, I took a deep breath, steeling myself for whatever news they would bring. 'The bronchoscopy showed that

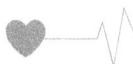

the lung tissue and bronchus are in reasonably good condition,' one doctor began, a glimmer of hope creeping into his voice. 'However, we need to address the collapsed bronchus that isn't allowing air through to his left lung.'

I felt a flicker of relief at the good news, but it was quickly overshadowed by what came next.

'We will discuss this with the surgical team, develop a plan, and then we will inform you of the outcome,' the doctor concluded, offering a small reassuring smile before they left the room.

As the door clicked shut, the pressure of uncertainty seemed to settle even heavier on my chest. Tee and I sat there in silence for a few moments, processing what had just been said. It felt like the calm before the storm.

Later that evening, we were called back to meet with the team. My pulse quickened as we made our way down the hospital corridors, each step echoing in the quiet night. I felt the tension build with each passing moment, a sense of impending dread settling deep within me.

We entered the small conference room where the surgical team was already waiting. The chairs felt too hard, too cold, as we sat down, bracing ourselves for the news we

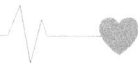

were about to receive. My mind raced with questions, fears, and a thousand possible outcomes, but the only thing I could focus on was the need to know what would happen next.

'We've spoken to the surgical team, and we believe Lion will need another surgery,' the doctor announced.

The air rushed from my lungs as I struggled to process his words. 'Another surgery?' I whispered, disbelief flooding my voice. 'He hasn't even woken up from the first one—how can you possibly... go back in?' A sob escaped me, raw and broken. Tee held me tightly, his own pain evident in the way his body shook.

The doctor placed a gentle hand on my shoulder, his expression sympathetic. 'We understand how overwhelming this is,' he said softly. 'Due to the prolonged time on the ventilator, which can have its own impacts, we want to get Lion off of it as soon as possible. We're recommending surgery within the next 24 to 48 hours. It's a difficult decision, but we believe it's the best course of action to help him breathe independently. The surgeon will attempt to stitch up the clamped area of the main bronchus, and in doing that, we hope to resolve the issue.'

I looked at Tee, my heart pounding with a mix of fear and confusion.

'Do you have any questions?' the doctor asked gently.

We both shook our heads, still in shock from the conversation. Words failed us as we grappled with the immensity of what lay ahead.

As the doctors left the room, I leaned my head against Tee's shoulder, my tears soaking through his shirt. The smell of antiseptic lingered in the air, mixing with the sterile scent of the hospital, a harsh reminder of where we were. 'Please stop crying, babe,' he whispered, his voice thick with emotion. 'Lion is a fighter. He has come this far. He needs us to be strong, too.'

I felt the warmth of his comfort, but the heaviness in my heart remained. It was true; Lion had shown remarkable strength, battling through every challenge thrown his way, but the fear gripping me was relentless. A shadow that loomed larger with each passing moment.

That night, we sat by Lion's bedside, our voices low as we whispered encouragements into the stillness of the room. The rhythmic beeping of the monitors was a constant reminder of his fragile state, and my heart broke every

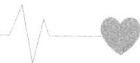

time I looked at his tiny body, so still and vulnerable. We held his tiny hand, our fingers enveloping his, willing him to feel our love and support. Hours stretched into an agonising eternity, and eventually, fatigue settled over us like a heavy blanket.

When we finally returned to the accommodation, each step felt heavy, as though the fullness reality pressed down on us like an unbearable burden. We trudged through the door, the emptiness of the space echoing our distress.

Inside, Milo and Hugo, came running up to us, their innocent smiles piercing through the gloom. Milo full of curiosity, tugged on my arm, his bright eyes wide with hope. 'Mummy, when can Lion come home?'

'Soon, darling,' I whispered, wrapping my arms around him tightly, desperately trying to hide the anguish in my voice.

Hugo, ever the imaginative one, held up a colourful drawing he'd made. 'I made this for Lion,' he said proudly, his little face beaming with excitement. It was a crayon-rendered dinosaur, bright green with a goofy grin.

'That's amazing, sweetheart. He'll love it,' I replied, my voice cracking as I fought to maintain composure.

I hugged them closely, the warmth of their small bodies offering a flicker of comfort amidst the turmoil.

After we put the boys to bed, Tee settled beside me, his eyes fixed on a point somewhere far beyond the walls of our room. 'Listen, babe,' he said, his voice low but resolute, breaking the heavy silence. 'If this second surgery will save Lion, then we'll do it. We've come too far to lose hope now. He needs us to believe in him.'

His words struck a chord deep within me, a bittersweet blend of hope and fear. I nodded, though my heart felt like a tangled mess, caught in a constant battle between dread and optimism. As I lay in bed that night, tears slipped silently down my cheeks, each droplet carrying a multitude of what-ifs circling relentlessly in my mind, but in the stillness, I clung to the flicker of hope Tee's words had reignited within me. Lion was a fighter, a tiny warrior in a world far too large for him, and we would fight alongside him, step by agonising step, for as long as it took. Together, we would navigate the storm, ready to face whatever came next, knowing our love was the bulwark we all needed.

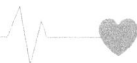

CHAPTER 17

The Unexpected Miracle

On the day of the second surgery, as Tee and I walked through the hospital to drop off Milo and Hugo at the hospital school, I felt a wave of mixed emotions: anticipation intertwined with dread. That day was crucial for Lion; it was the day of his second surgery. My heart raced as we approached the main entrance of the hospital, and I exchanged a brief, knowing glance with Tee, who stood beside me, holding onto Milo and Hugo. We were caught in a whirlwind of emotions, shifting from fleeting moments of hope to overwhelming fear.

The medical team had been working tirelessly to stabilise Lion's breathing, trying every possible intervention to avoid surgery. Despite their best efforts, however, nothing seemed to offer a lasting solution. His breathing remained

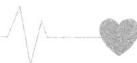

laboured, a constant reminder that surgery might be the only path forward to give him the chance he needed to survive.

A heavy weight settled in my chest as Tee and I both braced ourselves for the uncertainty that loomed ahead. We were about to sign the paperwork for Lion's surgery, yet it felt as though we were stepping off a precipice into a reality I wasn't ready to face. Numbness overtook me, and I moved through the motions as if I were trapped in a dream. I had left my phone and bag behind, taking only myself, Tee, and the kids with me.

While Tee branched off to the reception to collect our second key for our hospital accommodation, I stepped into the lift, the cool metal walls enclosing me as it ascended towards the Paediatric Intensive Care Unit, each floor passing by in a blur as I steeled myself for what awaited. My heart was heavy with anticipation, but I kept moving, each step bringing me closer to Lion. My only focus was being with him, even as my mind raced with all the unknowns that lay ahead.

I stepped out of the lift and the sterile smell of the hospital enveloped me. I walked down the corridor, the sounds of medical equipment and hushed voices echoing around me. Dr London, Lion's surgeon, approached. He seemed

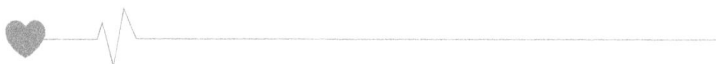

surprised to see me back so soon after leaving so late the previous night, but there was something else in his eyes, a flicker of relief, perhaps even of hope.

'Hello,' he greeted me warmly, stopping a few feet away. 'How are you holding up today?'

I took a shaky breath, the knot of anxiety in my stomach tightening. 'Not too good,' I admitted, my voice barely above a whisper as I struggled to meet his gaze. The heaviness in my heart made each word feel like an effort.

He paused for a moment, and his expression softened. 'I just came from a meeting with the team,' he began, his tone carefully light, surprising me with its unexpected ease. 'And there's been a bit of an update.' He took a breath and locked eyes with me. 'We might not be going in for the second surgery after all. There was an improvement in his airway overnight.'

The words didn't immediately register. Confusion washed over me as I stared at him, my mind spinning 'I—wait, what? Are you saying... Lion doesn't need the surgery?'

'Correct,' he replied, a smile breaking through the tension. 'Things have changed. His condition improved

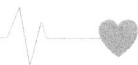

significantly enough overnight that we feel surgery can be postponed for now.'

I felt my knees go weak as the weight of his words slowly sunk in. Overwhelmed, I struggled to find my voice, feeling as if I'd been handed an impossible gift.

'Can I hug you, please?' The words spilled out before I could think.

Dr London nodded, surprise flickering across his face just before I wrapped my arms around him and held on with every ounce of strength I had. It wasn't merely a thank you; it was a release of all the terror and tension I had been carrying, every silent prayer whispered into the night, every fear kept buried deep within. Tears streamed down my face as I clung to him, feeling a shroud dissolve for the first time in what felt like forever. Dr London's hand rested gently on my back, patting me softly as his voice became a soothing murmur. 'Hang in there. The team will be with you soon to explain everything in detail.'

He eventually pulled away and offered me a reassuring smile as he turned to leave. I felt my entire body relax. It was as if I could finally take a deep breath. Just then, the lift doors opened, and Tee stepped out, his face etched with worry. As he approached, I couldn't help but smile through my tears, the hope of the moment shimmering brightly between us.

'Is everything okay?' Tee asked, his eyes searching mine for answers.

'It's better than okay,' I replied, my voice trembling with relief. 'Lion doesn't need the surgery after all!'

Tee's expression shifted from concern to sheer disbelief. His brows lifted in surprise. 'Really? That's incredible!'

I nodded, unable to contain my joy any longer. 'It really is! The doctors said there was an improvement in his airway overnight. We have more time.'

He wrapped me in his arms, holding me tightly as the shadow of our worries began to lift. In that moment, I knew we were in this together, ready to face whatever challenges lay ahead, anchored by the flicker of hope that had been reignited within us.

'Thank goodness,' Tee whispered, his forehead resting gently against mine, our breaths mingling in the charged air of the PICU. 'Our warrior is fighting.' He paused, his gaze locking with mine 'Let's go see our son.'

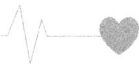

We made our way into the PICU, our hands tightly intertwined. As we stepped through the double doors, a sense of reverence washed over us, grounding us amidst the flood of emotions. Each step felt lighter, buoyed by the glimmering faith that had ignited in our hearts. We leaned over Lion's bed, watching in awe as his chest rose and fell. Each breath was a miracle, a testament to his strength and resilience. Although the rollercoaster of our journey wasn't over—his airway would still need vigilant monitoring, and the spectre of future surgery loomed large—that moment was a reprieve, a chance to pause and soak in the preciousness of life.

We settled into our chairs by Lion's side, our fingers gently stroking his tiny hand. 'You're doing so well, my warrior,' I whispered, the words dripping with all the love and encouragement I could muster. The machines around us beeped softly, a symphony of hope rather than dread. For once, they didn't heighten my anxiety; instead, they served as a quiet reminder of how incredibly precious every breath, every heartbeat, truly was.

Tee stepped out of the PICU for a moment to gather some essentials and send them back to our accommodation, leaving me alone with Lion. I watched him sleep for hours, the rhythmic hum of the machines becoming a lullaby in the sterile environment, silently pleaded for a miracle,

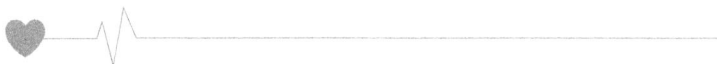

wishing I could trade places with him, feeling utterly helpless. Just then, Lion's bedside nurse approached. With a kind expression she said softly, 'The team would like to meet with you to discuss the plan for Lion.'

My heart raced at the thought of more discussions, more decisions. I took a shaky breath and leaned over to press a kiss on Lion's forehead, feeling the warmth of his skin against my lips before following the nurse down the corridor.

As I entered the conference room, I was met by a sea of professionals: cardiologists, paediatric doctors and nurses, an airway specialist and members of the family support team. Each face was serious, and I felt a lump rise in my throat. The sheer number of specialists in the room sent my heart into overdrive. It must be serious, I thought, dread creeping in.

The cardiologist stepped forward first, his voice gentle 'Hello, how are you holding up?' he asked, his eyes filled with compassion and understanding.

I opened my mouth to respond, but the words caught in my throat. 'I'm... not too good,' I finally managed to whisper, my voice trembling. Tears welled in my eyes, and before I knew it, the floodgates opened. 'This is Lion's

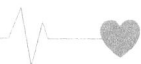

second week after his open-heart surgery, and I just... I just want to hear him call me Mama again,' I sobbed, each word heavy with emotion. 'He's full of life, always running around, chasing after his brothers, fighting for his toys, and running to me whenever he sees me. He calls out 'Mama' for everything.' My voice cracked as I continued, 'We miss him. Our entire family is going through this with him.'

The cardiologist nodded thoughtfully, allowing my words to settle in the room before he replied, 'From a cardiac perspective, Lion is doing fantastically. His heart is healing just as we hoped it would.' He paused, giving me a moment to absorb the good news. 'However,' he continued, his tone shifting, 'we need to address his breathing difficulties so we can help him wake up and start breathing on his own.'

Then, the airway specialist stepped forward, his demeanour compassionate. 'Lion will likely need a stent procedure to help open his airway,' he explained, his voice steady. A stent procedure involves inserting a small tube, called a stent, into a narrowed or blocked passageway in the body, such as a blood vessel or airway. The stent is designed to keep the passage open, allowing for improved blood flow or airflow,' he continued.

'In Lion's case, which is airway management, a stent can help maintain an open airway for him. The procedure typically involves placing the stent through a flexible tube, such as a bronchoscope, which is inserted into the airway. Once in position, the stent expands to hold the airway open, providing relief and facilitating better breathing.

'Stents can be temporary or permanent, depending on the patient's needs and the underlying condition being treated. Typically, these stents are custom made for each patient, and the waiting time is usually around three weeks.'

Three more weeks? Panic surged through me at the thought. 'Does that mean... Lion will stay on the ventilator all that time?' I asked, my voice trembling as tears streamed down my cheeks.

The doctor placed a comforting hand on my shoulder, his expression empathetic. 'We understand the urgency,' he reassured me, 'and fortunately, we do have a spare stent on hand. It was custom ordered for another child who no longer needs it. We believe this stent could work for Lion, allowing us to do the procedure much sooner.'

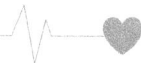

I blinked in disbelief, my heart racing with a mix of hope and fear. 'So, he might not have to wait weeks? This could happen soon?'

'Exactly,' the airway specialist affirmed, a hint of a smile breaking through the seriousness of the moment. 'We'll move quickly to get everything in place. Our priority is to ensure Lion can breathe on his own as soon as possible.'

As I absorbed the news, the fog of uncertainty began to lift, replaced by the spark of hope that had been so elusive. I clung to it, ready to face whatever came next for my brave little warrior.

As I sat there absorbing every detail of the conversation, I felt utterly drained, exhausted mentally and emotionally down to my very core. I looked up at the doctor, my voice barely a whisper, thick with all of the hope and fear tangled up in my heart. 'Please... please, do everything you can to save my Lion,' I managed to say. The plea hung heavily in the quiet room.

'We will,' the doctor replied with genuine warmth, his eyes steady, his words full of reassurance. Each member of the team nodded with quiet resolve before leaving to prepare for the procedure. Alone in the room, I realised

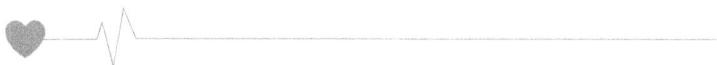

I needed my family by my side. My fingers shook as I dialled Tee's number, and he picked up almost at once.

'Tee, can you bring Milo and Hugo here? I want them to see Lion before the procedure, before we take the next step,' I said, my voice quivering.

A short while later, I returned to Lion's bedside, watching him as he lay surrounded by the rhythmic hum of machines. Those machines were his lifeline, yet they reminded me just how fragile he was. When Tee arrived with Milo and Hugo, all three of them stopped in the cubicle entrance, taking in the sight of their brother hooked up to tubes, his tiny body so still. Their expressions shifted from curiosity to worry, a look I'd never seen on their young faces before.

Milo stepped closer, his voice a hushed whisper. 'Mummy, why isn't Lion waking up?'

I knelt beside him, brushing his hair back gently. 'Lion is sleeping, sweetheart,' I said softly, my voice trembling slightly despite my best effort to keep it steady. 'But he's strong, and soon, he'll wake up and play with you again, just like always.'

The words seemed to reassure them. They nodded and drifted slowly to the play area set up by the kind-hearted

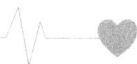

play specialist who'd been with us throughout our journey, finding ways to bring light and distraction for Milo and Hugo during the endless hospital hours.

The medical team returned a while later, carrying a stack of paperwork with carefully detailed terms and risks. Tee and I sat down and went over every word, signing each page with a mix of hope and caution, reminding us that Lion was strong all the while, —that he'd come this far, and he'd keep fighting.

As the team prepared to take him to the theatre, Tee and I shared a long, silent look, our hands tightly clasped as we tried to steady ourselves for what lay ahead. We watched as they wheeled him down the hall, his tiny body on the gurney, and then the door swung closed, leaving us in the silence.

'I think we should take Milo and Hugo for lunch,' Tee suggested, gently placing a hand on my shoulder. I nodded, realising he was right. The boys needed a sense of normalcy, and maybe we did, too.

We found a small café nearby and did our best to lift the boys' spirits, laughing over their stories and encouraging their wild imaginings, but every few moments, I'd catch

Tee's gaze across the table, both of us holding the same silent question: What's happening with Lion right now?

After lunch, we took Milo and Hugo to a nearby park. They ran ahead, their laughter ringing out, blissfully unaware of the shadow of worry that had settled over us. Their energy, their innocence—it reminded us of the resilience of children, the way they found joy even in the darkest moments.

Then, my phone rang. I froze, glancing at the screen. It was Dr Ron, Lion's airway specialist. My heart thudded as I answered. 'Hello?'

'Hi,' he began, his tone gentle. 'I wanted to let you know that Lion's procedure went smoothly. He did incredibly well. The stent is in place, and it's working as we hoped. He'll be returning to the PICU soon to continue his recovery.'

A wave of relief washed over me, leaving me breathless. I hadn't realised just how tense I'd been, holding my breath, waiting. 'Thank you. Thank you so much, Dr Ron,' I said, my voice thick with gratitude.

After I hung up, I turned to Tee, barely able to contain the surge of joy in my chest. 'He made it through,' I whispered,

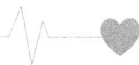

as if speaking it aloud might make it disappear. 'Lion made it. The procedure was a success.'

Tee's face broke into a smile, his eyes brimming with relief. He pulled me into a tight hug, both of us holding on as if to seal the moment of hope and triumph. We shared the news with Milo and Hugo, who burst into cheers, their innocent joy amplifying our own relief. To them, their little brother was safe; that was all they needed to know.

Tee decided to take Milo and Hugo back to the accommodation, giving me a chance to spend some time alone with Lion. I hugged them all tightly before returning to the PICU, feeling drawn to my son, my little warrior.

When I entered the room and saw him lying there, a mixture of peace and strength in his tiny frame, I felt an overwhelming surge of gratitude. I pulled a chair close to his bed and took his little hand in mine. I stroked his fingers softly, leaning close to whisper, 'You did it, my brave Lion. You're so strong, so resilient. We're all here, cheering you on, loving you every second.'

As I sat there, I felt the warmth of hope settle over me, a reminder that no matter the obstacles ahead, we would face them together. It was our small victory, a chance

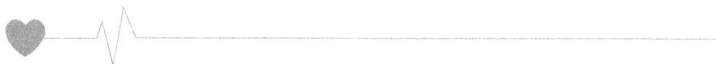

to breathe, to hold on to each other, and to cherish the miracle we'd just received.

I left the hospital later that day, a newfound calm replacing the fear that had gripped me so often. Yes, uncertainty still lingered — there were no guarantees on our journey — but for the first time, I felt as if we'd been given a gift, a break in the storm, a chance to gather strength.

As I walked back to the accommodation, I thought about the medical team's careful planning, the successful procedure, and the fierce resilience of my little Lion. In that moment, I allowed myself to simply feel grateful for the unexpected blessing we'd been given and the hope that would carry us forward.

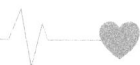

CHAPTER 18

Our Second Home

Life in the hospital became our new reality after Lion's heart surgery. The sterile scent of antiseptic hung in the air, and the constant hum of machinery filled every corner, yet it was the rhythmic beeps of the monitors that really became our daily soundtrack. Our lives shifted, adapted, and we found ourselves establishing a fragile routine within a world of uncertainty. Navigating hospital corridors, attending meetings with doctors, and taking care of Milo and Hugo while remaining fully present for Lion's recovery became second nature. Amidst the highs and lows, we managed to find a rhythm, piecing together moments of stability within the chaos of Lion's recovery journey.

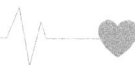

Just as we had started to adjust, another devastating blow shattered the fragile balance we had fought so hard to build. My father's health took a sudden and dramatic turn for the worse. The hospital, which had been the epicentre of our fight for Lion's life, would soon become the battleground for another precious soul, holding both my son's and my father's futures in its hands.

We found refuge in a small family room provided by the hospital, a four-bed space that, despite its simplicity, became our sanctuary amidst the storm. The room held fragments of our lives, offering some semblance of normalcy in the chaos: a few of the boys' favourite toys, a worn blanket that reminded us of home and the faint, comforting scent of the lavender sachet we always kept by the window.

In that small, cluttered space, Tee, the children and I huddled together, holding tightly to one another. We had no choice but to cling to the bond of family, navigating through each day filled with tension, worry and exhaustion. The outside world may have continued, but within those walls, we lived in a bubble of uncertainty, finding strength in each other, determined to keep our family together no matter the challenges we faced.

My father had been staying with us at the hospital accommodation, offering his steady presence and quiet support as he stood by Lion and the rest of us. His calm and unwavering love had been a comfort through the chaos, grounding us as we navigated one hurdle after another. While his health had always been a concern, we hadn't anticipated what would come.

It began innocently enough. He started feeling unwell, but we assumed it was just the weight of the stress taking its toll. The constant worry over Lion's recovery had begun to wear on him. He mentioned that his little toe was bothering him, a minor discomfort at first that we dismissed as something trivial, but when he finally mentioned it again, we decided to have it looked at. A visit to the general practitioner revealed what the doctor was thought was a simple case of athlete's foot, a common fungal condition. He was given a course of antibiotics and antifungal cream, and we believed that would be the end of it, but it wasn't. What we thought was a minor issue soon escalated in ways we never could have imagined, but before he could complete the antibiotic course, his symptoms rapidly worsened. He went from being the vibrant, supportive father able to brighten any room to a shadow of his former self. His usual warmth and liveliness seemed to disappear, his laughter became scarce and his energy dwindled. It was as if a light inside him

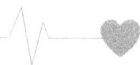

had dimmed, and an unshakable sense of dread began to settle in my heart.

It was hard to reconcile that the man who had been our pillar of strength now needed our support as much as Lion did. The weight of seeing two of my loved ones battling their own vulnerabilities under the same roof was overwhelming, and we leaned even more into each other. The family room became our shelter in which we tried to recreate a semblance of normalcy in the face of uncertainty, but the feeling of helplessness lingered, with each day becoming a battle not only for Lion's health but also for my father's.

One evening, I returned to our accommodation after spending hours by Lion's bedside. Following his stent procedure, he'd shown signs of improvement, and for the first time in days, I felt a glimmer of relief. I opened the door and found my father resting in his bed, looking more fragile than I'd ever seen him.

'Hello, Dad,' I greeted softly, hoping he'd comfort in my presence.

'Hello, Ezy,' he fondly replied, his voice weak and wavering.

I noticed a tired pallor in his face, and a worry that had been growing inside me started to intensify. 'Dad, I really think we should go to the hospital again and get you checked out,' I said, carefully watching his expression.

'No, no,' he insisted with a slight wave of his hand. 'I'm recovering. You just need to rest, Ezy.' He was stubborn, always wanting to shield me, even now.

'Please, Dad,' I urged, my voice edged with worry. 'I think it's important. I'd feel better if we went.'

He looked at me for a long moment, perhaps realising just how worried I was, and finally nodded, though he added with a gentle smile, 'All right, but let's be quick. You need to rest, too. You've been through so much. I need you strong.'

'Okay, Dad,' I replied softly, but the urgency in my heart didn't ease.

I took him to the hospital, thinking it would be a routine check-up, a chance to ease my concerns. Tee stayed back at the accommodation with Milo and Hugo, managing everything in my absence. I expected the doctors to suggest some additional rest, perhaps an adjustment to

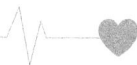

his medication or a simple remedy for his fatigue, but the reality awaiting us was nothing of the sort.

After a long wait and several tests, a doctor approached us with a sombre expression. 'Your father has developed severe complications from diabetes,' he explained. 'It appears diabetic neuropathy has affected his toe, and the infection is serious. We're going to need to admit him immediately, and surgery may be necessary.'

The words hit me like a punch to the chest. I felt as if the air had been stolen from the room. 'How… how can this be happening?' I murmured, trying to process it. My mind raced, consumed by a storm of emotions and questions.

I looked over at my father, hoping to find some reassurance in his expression, but he looked away, almost resigned, his normally spirited gaze replaced by something more fragile. In that moment, the weight of my circumstances crashed down upon me. I wasn't just Lion's mother fighting for his life anymore; I was a daughter watching my father's health unravel before my eyes. It felt impossible, like being pulled into two separate worlds of heartbreak, each one demanding more of me than I felt capable of giving.

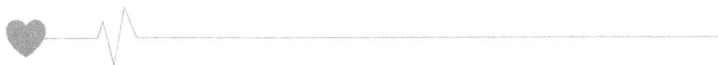

After my dad was admitted, I returned to our accommodation, numb and exhausted. As soon as I walked in, I broke down, my shoulders shaking under the immense pressure of everything I'd been holding in.

'I don't know if I can do this,' I whispered to Tee, tears streaming down my cheeks. 'What if… what if something happens to him? How could I bear it?'

Tee wrapped his arms around me, his embrace the only anchor I had left. 'You don't have to do it alone. We'll figure this out together, we always do,' he said, his voice steady, grounding.

Even with his arms around me, the hospital—once a place of hope for Lion—felt suffocating, heavy with the needs of two of the people I loved most. The despair and the feeling of being torn apart, left me feeling hollow, and in that moment, it felt as though the walls were closing in, and the heaviness of it all would swallow me whole.

The days ahead turned into a blurred cycle of hospital corridors, beeping machines and quiet tears shed in the shadows. I was constantly moving between Lion's bedside and my father's room, with Tee and I taking turns by their sides. Our lives were split between supporting Lion through his fragile recovery and comforting my

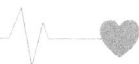

father through his own medical battle. All the while, we somehow tried to keep things steady for Milo and Hugo, who were caught up in the storm of uncertainty.

I'll never forget those quiet moments when I sat alone, finally still, my face in my hands, wondering how much more I could handle. My heart felt torn in two, stretched impossibly thin between Lion's needs and my father's. I was exhausted to my core, yet each time I felt like breaking, the thought of my family kept me going.

One evening, I sat beside Lion, who was finally sleeping peacefully. His little chest rose and fell in a steady rhythm, and for the first time, his colour seemed a bit better. I leaned back in my chair, closed my eyes and tried to centre myself, hoping for a moment of peace in the chaos.

The door creaked open, and I felt a hand rest gently on my shoulder. It was Tee. 'Hey, babe,' he said softly, his voice full of warmth and concern. 'How are you holding up?'

I opened my eyes and looked at him, feeling the gravity of everything pressing down on me. 'I don't know, Tee,' I whispered. 'It feels like I'm losing control. Lion needs me, but so does my dad. I don't know how to be there for both without… without falling apart.'

Tee knelt down beside me, his gaze unwavering, his voice soft. 'You're doing everything you can,' he said, his hand tightening around mine. 'It's okay to feel overwhelmed. Just... let's take it one moment at a time. That's all we need to get through this.'

I felt a surge of gratitude, his words filling the empty spaces in my heart with a sense of calm. I nodded, took a shaky breath, and for a moment, the cloud lifted just a little.

Through the heartache, a glimmer of hope began to emerge. Though My father's initial diagnosis seemed grim. My father began to show small signs of improvement. His familiar sense of humour started to peek through, and I'd see flashes of his old self, the father who had always been there for me, now fighting his own battle to stay by my side.

One day, his doctor pulled me aside with a reassuring smile. 'Your father is making progress. The surgery went well, and he's responding to treatment. We're optimistic he'll make a full recovery.'

Relief washed over me in a wave so strong it left me feeling weak. I returned to his bedside, and we exchanged a silent look of shared relief and determination. With his

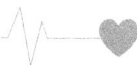

recovery now on the horizon, I felt a renewed sense of strength and focus, and I could turn more fully to Lion, pouring everything I had left into his healing.

Later that day, as I entered Lion's room, I took his tiny hand in mine and whispered a promise to him and to my father, a promise to be strong for them both, to carry hope through every challenge that lay ahead. Although our journey was far from over, in that moment, I felt a sense of readiness. I was bolstered by the love surrounding me and the small victories that reminded me to keep going, one step at a time.

Lion was a true warrior, inching his way through recovery. Day by day, he began to come off sedation and the strong painkillers that had kept him comfortable. Each slight movement, each flicker of awareness, felt monumental, a cherished sign that he was coming back to us.

One day, as I was with Milo and Hugo in the play area, trying to keep things light for them and give them a break from the intensity of the hospital, one of Lion's bedside nurses hurried in, her face radiant with excitement. 'Come quick! Lion's opening his eyes,' she exclaimed, her voice bright with joy.

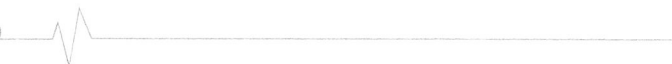

My heart leapt, and I raced to his side, my pulse hammering. There he was, my brave little Lion. His eyes fluttered open, his gaze unfocused but slowly finding me. I leaned in close, feeling every emotion surge at once.

'Hey, love,' I whispered, my voice choked with awe, 'can you see me?'

His eyes met mine, and though they were heavy with the remnants of sedation, there was a spark there, a quiet recognition, and a faint, babbling sound escaped his lips. He reached his tiny hand toward me, a motion so delicate yet so strong that it felt as if he were grasping my very soul. He tried to say something, and the soft babble that came out sounded almost like 'Mama.'

Tears streamed down my face as I took his hand, overcome by the flood of emotions. 'Yes, my little warrior, it's Mama,' I whispered, clutching his hand tightly. 'You're so strong, and I'm right here with you. I love you more than anything.'

From that moment, Lion continued his slow, steady journey back to us, and every step forward felt like a gift. He began to fully wake from his long sedation, his eyes brighter each day, but with the sedation wearing off, new challenges appeared. His body, having been so still for

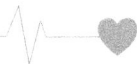

so long, needed to learn to move again. His muscles had weakened, and even the smallest movements took all of his effort.

The physiotherapist came to help rebuild his strength, guiding him through exercises to stretch and move his limbs. Watching him struggle to lift his little arms, knowing those movements used to be effortless, was gut-wrenching.

'Come on, Lion,' I cheered softly as the physiotherapist gently encouraged him to wiggle his toes. 'You can do it, my love. Just a little more—let's see those wiggling toes!'

Lion's determination was pure and fierce. His brow furrowed in concentration, and with a small grunt of effort, his toes moved, then his arms lifted slightly. His eyes lit up with pride, and a joyful sound escaped him, a beautiful blend of laughter and excitement.

'Yes! Look at you! You're amazing!' I cried, my heart swelling with pride as I watched his tiny victories unfold.

With each passing day, he fought back harder, reclaiming his strength bit by bit. I could see the fire in him, an indomitable spirit that reminded me of how deeply his name suited him. He was my Lion, strong and unbreakable, roaring back to life.

Every day with Lion brought a new milestone: lifting his tiny arm, wiggling his legs, even managing to sit up with a little help. Each small achievement felt monumental, and the team of nurses and physiotherapists rallied around him, marvelling at his progress.

'Lion, you're our superstar!' one nurse beamed, gently pinching his cheek. 'Look at you go, little warrior.'

Lion giggled, a sound so pure it seemed to fill the entire room, lifting the spirits of everyone around him. For so long, the halls had echoed with the sterile hum of machines and quiet, tense whispers. Now, his laughter was a reminder of the beautiful, innocent life we were fighting for.

Then came the day I had been holding my breath for: the removal of his breathing tube. It had been both his lifeline and the very symbol of his struggle, tethering him to the machines that had sustained him through the most critical moments. As the tube came out, the nurses carefully watching, I held my breath alongside Lion. He took a tentative first breath, then another, his small chest

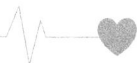

rising and falling without the aid of any machine. It was a miracle in motion.

Tears filled my eyes as I watched him breathe freely for the first time since his surgery. I had longed for that moment, a sign that his body was strong enough to sustain itself, that he was beginning to recover. It felt like a promise of life beyond the hospital walls.

Without the barriers of tubes and monitors, I could finally hold him close. I gathered him gently in my arms, feeling his warmth against me. His wide eyes glazed up, sparkling with a newfound light, his face breaking into a joyful smile. Every time I held him, it felt like reclaiming a part of the life we had before our whirlwind journey.

'Do you want to play with your toys?' I asked, reaching over to the small collection we had accumulated at his bedside. I held up his favourite, a small, stuffed grey dinosaur with a friendly smile.

Lion's eyes widened. His little hand reached eagerly out. He pointed with delight, and I handed him the dinosaur. He clutched it tightly, bringing it to his face with the purest look of joy, his laughter ringing through the room.

'*Roar!*' he pretended, his small voice full of glee as he shook the dinosaur with all his might.

The medical team gathered, smiling and cheering him on. Those were the moments that reminded me how much he had endured and how far he had come. Slowly, the room began to fill with light, laughter and echoes of hope.

Lion's recovery continued to defy expectations. Soon, he was strong enough to be moved out of the Paediatric Intensive Care Unit to the Paediatric Cardiac Care Unit, a step-down unit where children were still monitored closely but didn't require intensive, round-the-clock intervention. The move felt monumental, like the beginning of a new chapter. Just 48 hours later, his strength was stable enough for yet another move to a regular ward with fewer restrictions, a place where children could play, laugh and begin to fully heal.

Each transfer was a significant step forward, a visible testament to his resilience and strength. I watched him gain not only physical strength but also a glimmer of his playful spirit. Little by little, his laugh returned, his eyes sparkled with curiosity, and he began reaching for toys, exploring the room around him as if he were seeing the world anew. Every smile, every burst of laughter felt like a piece of our family coming back together.

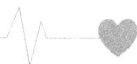

As Lion continued his recovery, I saw in him the unbreakable spirit of a true warrior, a child who had faced a battle and come through stronger, brighter and ready for all the joy yet to come.

With Lion's progress in recovery, the possibility of bringing him home seemed closer each day. Conversations with the doctors became laced with hints of discharge. The very thought of having him back in our home, watching him play alongside his brothers and enjoying simple family moments without hospital walls felt like a long-lost dream finally come true.

One night, as Tee and I lay in bed, the veil of exhaustion pressing down on us, he turned to me with a faint smile. 'Can you imagine what it'll be like when he's finally home?'

I felt my chest warm and my heart swell. 'He'll be running around, driving us crazy with his boundless energy like he used to. I can't wait to see him back to his old, playful self,' I replied, laughing softly at the thought. We lay there, letting ourselves get lost in a dream of normalcy, holding onto it like a lifeline that pulled us through the endless days of waiting and uncertainty.

The excitement grew with each day as Lion continued to amaze everyone with his progress. His laughter echoed in the halls of the ward, and the light in his eyes shone brighter, as if he, too, knew he was on the brink of freedom.

Finally, the much-anticipated day arrived. As I dressed him, his little hands clutched his favourite dinosaur. The nurses who had become like family gathered around, their faces alight with joy and pride. They had watched over him with the same love and dedication they would give their own, and now they were there to send him off with all the encouragement in the world.

'You did it, Lion! You're going home!' one nurse said, bending down to his level and grinning widely.

Lion's eyes sparkled as he bounced on his feet, his little body practically vibrating with excitement. 'Mama!' he babbled, pointing eagerly toward the door with a delighted squeal as if to say, 'Let's go!' His smile stretched wide across his face, his joy contagious.

I glanced around the room, my heart a chaotic mix of emotions. The space had been our battleground, a place where every beep of a machine, every hurried step of a nurse, every whispered prayer had become the backdrop of our lives. Now, it was just a room. I would always hear

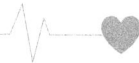

the hum of the machines in my mind, but in that moment, the memories softened, fading as we stepped into the new reality.

Tears welled in my eyes, spilling over as I hugged each nurse, each doctor and every staff member who had cared for Lion and held our hands through our journey. They had been our pillars, and saying goodbye was harder than I could have imagined.

With Lion in my arms, his dinosaur clutched tightly in his little fist, we took our final steps down the hospital corridor. The halls that had once felt cold and daunting now seemed to shine with a lightness I hadn't noticed before. The doors opened, and fresh air flooded over us, a simple pleasure that felt like freedom itself.

CHAPTER 19

Homecoming and Recovery

Stepping outside felt surreal, as if I were waking from a long, heavy dream. The hospital's sterile walls and fluorescent lights faded behind us, replaced by a world brimming with colour, light and possibility. The crisp air filled my lungs as I held Lion close, his laughter bubbling up like music, his tiny fingers stretching eagerly towards the open sky. It was as if he could sense this was a moment of freedom, a step into a life he had only glimpsed through hospital windows and fading ceiling tiles.

Tee stood beside me, holding Milo's and Hugo's hands. He wrapped his free arm around my shoulders and pulled us close, his face a mirror of my own relief and

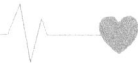

joy, a silent testament to everything we'd endured and finally overcome. We paused there, the five of us huddled together, feeling the burden of the journey lifting away. The months of sleepless nights, the anxious hours, the never-ending cycle of hope and fear—all of it melted, leaving only the pure, quiet joy of the moment.

I glanced down at Milo and Hugo, their faces glowing with wonder as they looked up at their baby brother. Their eyes sparkled with the innocence and excitement I hoped Lion would come to know; a childhood untouched by the shadows of medical wards. That was the life we had fought for, the life waiting for us on the other side of those hospital doors.

As we buckled Lion into his car seat, my heart raced with a mixture of joy and anticipation. Tee met my eyes, and in that moment, no words were needed. We both understood it was the start of something new, a chapter written with hope, healing and the strength we had found together. Milo and Hugo leaned in to say hello to their little brother, their voices brimming with excitement. It felt like our family was finally complete, whole and heading home, ready to embrace the life we'd dreamt of in countless hospital corridors.

'We're really going home, Lion,' Milo shouted, bouncing in his seat, eyes bright with joy. His voice rang through the car, a melody of hope that wrapped around each of us.

Beside him, Hugo reached over and gently held Lion's tiny hand. 'We missed you so much, Lion!' he said, his voice thick with emotion. They had struggled to understand why Lion had been in the hospital for so long, surrounded by machines and doctors, yet despite their confusion, they never stopped asking, 'When will he come home?' Now, their wait was finally over.

A lump rose in my throat as I took in the beautiful moment. Leaning over to Tee, I whispered, 'It's been a long road, but we're finally together again.'

He squeezed my hand, 'Yes,' he murmured, 'we made it.'

As we pulled out of the hospital parking lot, the sunlight poured through the car windows, illuminating the road ahead. A strange combination of hope and apprehension washed over me. While I was thrilled to finally have Lion home, a part of me still worried about his health, about the unknowns that lay ahead. The hospital, with all its fears, had become a place of safety where trained hands watched over him. Now, we were taking that responsibility into our own hands, a thought both empowering and daunting.

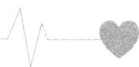

As I looked around at my family, at the joy in Milo's and Hugo's eyes, at Tee's reassuring smile, at Lion's quiet, peaceful face, I felt hope settle in my chest, warm and reassuring. Whatever lay ahead, we would face it together.

The entire drive was filled with Milo and Hugo's excited chatter as they animatedly recounted all the things Lion had 'missed' while he was in the hospital: their favourite cartoons, their new games and all the adventures they'd planned for him. Lion clutched his beloved dinosaur toy, babbling along as if he understood every word, as if he, too, knew he was heading back to the warmth and safety of home.

When we finally arrived, I felt a surge of emotion as I stepped inside, holding Lion close. The familiar scent of home wrapped around us, comforting and grounding. Tears pricked at my eyes as I looked around the living room, now filled with toys and memories waiting to be made. The space, once a sanctuary of laughter, had seen moments of despair, but now, it felt renewed, a place where we could start fresh, where Lion could grow strong and healthy.

Milo leaned over and whispered to Lion, 'We're going to show you everything! You're going to love it here!' I realised then that, despite the long and difficult journey that had brought us to that point, we were ready for a new chapter.

The first days at home were a whirlwind of adjustments. The medical team had left us with a long list of instructions on how to care for Lion, and I was determined to follow them to the letter. Every little cough, every small sigh, sent a shiver of anxiety through me, and I found myself constantly checking his breathing, even as he slept peacefully in his crib. I knew I had to let myself relax, to let go of some of the fear, but the instinct to protect him was overwhelming.

Tee and I quickly settled into a new routine, dividing the responsibilities of caring for our three children as we navigated the complexities of caring for a toddler with special health needs. 'I'll take the first shift with feedings and diaper changes,' I offered one morning, doing my best to keep my voice steady.

Tee nodded, a glimmer of relief in his eyes. 'Sounds good. I'll take the next round.' He smiled and gave my shoulder a reassuring squeeze. 'We've got this together.'

There was something comforting in the rhythm of feedings and diaper changes, in the familiar tasks that anchored me amidst the swirl of emotions. With each day, I saw Lion

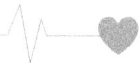

grow stronger, his cheeks regained a healthy blush. His eyes were bright and curious. Each small step forward felt like a victory, a reminder of how far we had come, but even as Lion thrived, I couldn't shake the shadows of our hospital experience. 'What if he gets sick again?' I often thought, a knot of anxiety tightening in my chest.

Friends and family rallied around us, offering their unwavering support. 'We can't wait to see him,' my sister Chloe said over the phone. Each visitor brought a sense of normalcy, a welcome distraction from the lingering fear, yet despite their presence, I struggled to relax, still haunted by the fragility of Lion's health.

As the days turned into weeks, we found our rhythm. I realised that Lion's recovery wasn't just about him; it was about our whole family. I made it my mission to create a home filled with love and laughter, determined to banish the shadow of hospital walls from our lives.

Lion began to flourish. His laughter, bright and infectious, filled our home like music, a promise of the future we had fought so hard for. Milo and Hugo quickly included him in their games, eager to show him their favourite toys and make him laugh. 'Come on, Lion, let's go play,' Milo would shout, beaming with excitement.

Those family moments, both big and small, became our new normal. I cherished every laugh, every shared smile, every quiet moment together. Our home, once a place of uncertainty, was now a sanctuary of healing and joy, yet even in these joyful moments, I remained acutely aware of the challenges still ahead. Doctor appointments loomed on the horizon, each one a fresh reminder of the unknowns that remained. As we prepared for the next check-up, I found solace in connecting with other parents who had walked similar paths. Their resilience, their unwavering hope, reminded me that we were not alone. 'It's tough, but we're making it,' one mother shared during a support group meeting. Her words, a reminder that we were part of a larger community of strength, comforted me.

During the follow-up appointments, I often sat in the waiting room surrounded by other parents who were clinging to their own fragile hopes. Some had bright, hopeful eyes; others looked exhausted, worn down by the weight of worry. There was a silent camaraderie in that room, a shared understanding of battles fought and fears closely held. A simple smile or nod from a fellow parent was enough to say, 'I know. I understand.'

But as our name was called and we stood to leave the room, that comforting sense of solidarity faded, replaced by the familiar tension that always seemed to accompany

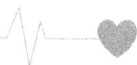

those moments. Tee's hand tightened on my shoulder as we walked into the doctor's office. My heart pounded, a strange mix of dread and anticipation knotting inside me.

The doctor examined Lion, carefully studying his chart, looking for signs of progress. Then, he looked up and smiled. 'He's doing remarkably well,' he said, his voice warm and reassuring. 'Lion is thriving.'

The relief was overwhelming. Tears filled my eyes as I turned to Tee, who looked as moved as I felt. We had fought so hard for that moment, had dreamt of hearing those words. 'We did it,' I whispered.

Tee smiled, his own voice soft. 'Yes, we did.'

As the weeks passed, our home continued to fill with joy and laughter. We embraced a routine, creating a stable environment where Lion could thrive. We shared family dinners, read bedtime stories, and went for walks together. Slowly, the shadow of our experiences began to lift, replaced by a sense of peace.

There were still setbacks, moments that reminded us of how fragile Lion's health was. When he had to be briefly admitted for fluid around his heart, I found myself reliving every nightmare from the NICU, but in those

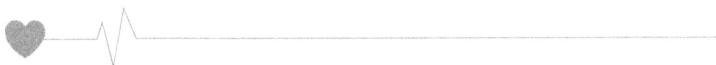

moments of darkness, Tee was there, a steady presence reminding me that it was okay to feel vulnerable, to lean on each other for strength.

Through every triumph and every setback, I learnt to find beauty in the present. Each day was a gift, each smile from Lion a reminder of the resilience that had carried us through. I cherished the simple joys that had bound us as a family, grateful for the love that had brought us to that moment.

One evening, after a day filled with laughter, I tucked Milo, Hugo and finally, Lion, into bed. I lay beside him, watching his peaceful face as he drifted off to sleep. His soft, steady breathing filled the room, and I felt a quiet gratitude wash over me, the weight of our journey settling into a sense of peace.

In that stillness, I realised that our journey hadn't only transformed Lion; it had reshaped us all. Tee and I had grown closer than ever, our shared experiences deepening the love that had sustained us through the hardest moments. We found strength in our vulnerability in the moments we had to lean on each other without reserve. The hardship had carved out a new space for empathy and resilience within us, qualities that now anchored our relationship in ways I hadn't imagined before.

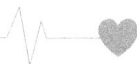

Milo and Hugo, too, had grown in ways I hadn't expected. They learned about love in its purest form, the kind that requires patience, sacrifice and celebration of the smallest milestones. They'd watched their baby brother fight against the odds, and in doing so, they'd learned the value of persistence, compassion, and the beauty of cherishing each moment. For children so young, they had developed an incredible awareness and empathy that would shape them for years to come.

And I was also changed. I had come to understand that real strength didn't mean facing everything alone; it meant knowing when to ask for help, when to let others carry you, when to lean into hope even when it seemed distant. Through sleepless nights, anxious waits, and joyful breakthroughs, I'd learnt to find power in vulnerability, to rely on the love and support around me. Above all, I had learnt to hold onto hope like a guiding light, allowing it to lead me even in the darkest times. From the darkest days in the hospital to the warmth and brightness of home, we had emerged stronger; our family bonded together by a love that had been tested and deepened.

As Lion continued to grow defying every hurdle, I knew our future was bright. The doctors marvelled at his progress. His sparkling eyes and hearty laugh were a testament to his resilience. 'He's a fighter, just like his mother,' Tee often said, his pride evident.

As I watched our little Lion thrive, I knew we had fought our battle together. We were a family forged in hope, our hearts entwined in a story of healing and love. It was just the beginning, a chapter of strength that would carry us forward to wherever life would lead us next.

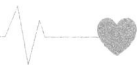

CHAPTER 20

Network of Support

As I sit here reflecting on the incredible support network that surrounded my family and me during the storm of Lion's first year, I'm amazed and deeply aware that we could not have made it through alone. I am eternally grateful for the unwavering support of Tee, my other children, Milo and Hugo, our family, our dear friends and the many healthcare professionals who played invaluable roles in our journey. Their support became an unbreakable pillar. It was a time filled with endless uncertainty and fear, a time that required more strength than I could have ever imagined. It was then I truly learned how the love and solidarity of those around me could make all the difference. When the pressing force of the world felt as if it would crush me, they lifted me up, reminding me that I was never alone on our journey.

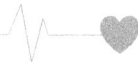

Tee was my rock, standing beside me through the sleepless nights, the hospital vigils, and the emotional rollercoaster that defined our days as parents to a heart warrior. There were moments I felt like I was drowning in worry, but Tee had this way of grounding me, a calm steadiness that kept me from being swept away. He knew just what to say, always with the quiet assurance that we were in this together. His presence became my anchor. Every hug, every gentle word, every reassuring touch soothed my frayed nerves, making me feel as if I could face whatever lay ahead. In Tee's eyes, I saw the strength we needed to keep going, and in his embrace, I found the courage to carry on.

I remembered how, as the days turned into weeks, my friends stepped up in ways I never could have imagined. They became my foundation, a source of love and encouragement that surrounded me during those long, lonely nights in the NICU, especially Willow and her husband Ethan, who offered unwavering support. They seemed to instinctively know what I needed. Willow's thoughtful gifts, like a 'hug in a jar' and handwritten notes filled with kind words, served as small but powerful reminders that I was loved and held in their thoughts. Those tokens meant the world to me, particularly during times when I felt completely alone in Lion's hospital room, with the soft beep of the monitors as my only companion.

One night stands out in my memory, a particularly dark evening when the shadow of despair loomed over me. I sat alone beside Lion, machines whirring softly in the background, struggling to keep my composure as fear of the unknown pressed in. Just then, my sister Olive called on a video call. I remember feeling warmth, an incredible sense of being cared for as we talked, and she encouraged me. Simple as it was, it was like a beacon that pulled me back from the edge, helping me feel loved and seen when I needed it most.

My friends, Clara and Ava, were pillars of strength during that time. They understood the depths of my struggles and never hesitated to reach out. Clara's empathetic nature meant she knew when to call just to listen. She gave me space to share my fears without judgement, reminding me it was okay to be overwhelmed and that I didn't need to wear a brave face all the time. Ava, who called every day to encourage me, often said, 'You're one of the strongest people I know, and Lion is so lucky to have you as his mum.' I remembered when I considered taking a gap year from university, and Ava encouraged me to take it if needed but reminded me I was almost at the finish line and that I was doing it not only for myself but for our family. Their words, their unwavering belief in me, became a safe space to express my worries and find solace.

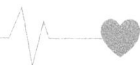

I remember one of the greatest things about one of my best friends, Camila, someone I had known since I was thirteen, back in secondary school. Despite living in a different country and not initially knowing the full extent of Lion's heart condition, she was nothing short of incredible. She made it her priority to check on me constantly. Whether it was through a simple message such as 'Take it easy, I love you' text or, a phone call, Camila never failed to show her care and concern.

When I eventually opened to her about Lion's heart condition, her support didn't falter. If anything, it deepened. She continued to check in on me regularly, her unwavering kindness reminding me that, even from miles away, I wasn't facing this journey alone.

Family, too, played an invaluable role. My parents and siblings—Chloe, Cora, Olive, Iris and Finn—rallied around me without hesitation. Chloe and my mother stepped in to help care for Lion during his hospital stays, allowing me precious time for my other children and my university and placement responsibilities. Their willingness to stand by me made an incredible difference, giving me the freedom to be present for all my children—Milo, Hugo and Lion—without feeling as if I were failing any of them. My brother Finn's encouragement was also unwavering. 'Your Lion deserves every fighting chance,' he reminded me. 'Never give up on him, and know I'm here for you.' His steadfastness was a comfort, a constant reminder that I had a solid foundation holding me up.

Additionally, Mamita, Tee's mom, emerged as another incredible source of strength during one of the most challenging times in our lives. With her warm smile and unwavering dedication, she took on the essential role of caring for Lion while I juggled my responsibilities at home and at university. Her presence brought a sense of calm to our chaotic household. Whenever she could, Mamita cooked delicious meals, filling our home with the comforting aromas of family recipes. She often tidied up, turning the chaos into order and alleviating the burdens of everyday life. Her thoughtful gestures and willingness to help not only kept our home running smoothly but also provided me with the invaluable gift of time—time I could devote to my family, university coursework and placement tasks without feeling overwhelmed.

With Mamita by my side, I felt a profound strain lift from my shoulders. She not only made sure that Lion, Milo and Hugo were cared for but also created a nurturing environment where I could breathe a little easier and focus on what truly mattered: my family, my studies, and supporting Lion's journey. Her love and support were

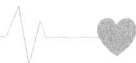

like a guiding light, leading me through the storm with a little more grace and a lot more hope.

Our neighbour, Daisy, who became like family over the years, was an unwavering source of support from the very beginning. She stepped in whenever she could, offering to take Milo and Hugo for a walk so I could focus on my university work without worry. She went above and beyond in so many ways, cleaning our outside bins, making sure they were set out for collection, and bringing them back once emptied, week after week, without fail. This small yet thoughtful gesture became a comforting part of our routine.

Her kindness extended to our children, too. She often surprised Milo and Hugo with little treats, bringing smiles to their faces and making them feel loved and cared for. She constantly checked in on us, offering words of encouragement and support, reminding us that we were not alone in our journey. Her warmth and dedication were a true blessing, a steady presence that lightened our load and reminded us of the kindness that surrounded us.

As a full-time student in my final year of social work, the guidance of my placement providers and university was equally invaluable. My supervisors and employers were understanding and accommodating in ways that went

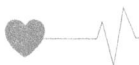

beyond what I could have expected. They recognised the emotional toll of my dual responsibilities as a mother and student and offered me flexibility whenever I needed to adjust my schedule.

My university tutors and dissertation supervisor were incredibly accommodating as well. I recall my dissertation supervisor offering sessions at my convenience, often late at night, just so I wouldn't feel overwhelmed. Friends from my course, though they didn't know all I was going through, checked in regularly. They shared resources, caught me up on missed lectures, and gave me the encouragement I needed to stay afloat.

One especially challenging hospitalisation left me feeling utterly exhausted, and during a catch-up meeting with my final-year practice educator, Leah, she insisted I take the week off. 'Turn off your phone, close your laptop, and rest,' she joked, but I could tell she meant it. Her words were a gift, a reminder that it was okay to rest, that people were rooting for me and wanting me to succeed in all parts of my life.

As Lion grew, facing milestone after milestone, the constant presence of my friends, family, university and placement providers remained steadfast. They celebrated every smile, every small victory, every glimmer of hope

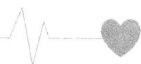

with us. Each milestone became a shared joy, a triumph that they cheered alongside us, no matter how small. With each laugh, each step forward, Lion showed us resilience, and together, we celebrated every precious moment.

Reflecting on that chapter of our lives, I now see that parenthood, especially with a child facing health challenges, is never a journey anyone should bear alone. The bonds we built, the community that rose up around us during our most trying times, stood as a testament to the power of love and friendship. I am eternally grateful for each person who stood by our side, offering their hands to hold and their hearts to share.

Even as we faced adversity, we found light in the love that surrounded us. The memories of their kindness continued to fuel my spirit, reminding me that, in the face of darkness, love and community truly are the greatest sources of strength. Together, we forged a path through that storm, finding hope in the depths of our connections, a hope that will forever be a part of our story.

CHAPTER 21

Reflection and Gratitude

As I sat quietly in the living room, the soft afternoon sunlight filtered through the windows, casting a warm, golden glow across the space. I watched Lion as he played with his toys, his giggles filling the air, a sweet melody that brought life to every corner. Each laugh was a small victory, a testament to his resilience, a reminder of how far we'd come. I was overcome with reflection and gratitude, humbled by the journey we'd taken together as a family. The road had been anything but smooth, yet each bump and turn had shaped us in ways I never imagined.

It was difficult to comprehend everything we have endured, from those early, agonising scans to the countless hours spent in hospital waiting rooms. I still vividly remembered those first appointments so clearly,

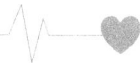

sitting in sterile rooms with cold, neutral walls, feeling the suffocating uncertainty that loomed, overwhelming and relentless. I would clutch my phone, anxiously waiting for any sign of hope, any news to break the silence. Each day was a reminder of life's fragility, of how quickly things could change, and yet, there we were, sitting in the warmth of our home, a place that had come to represent more than just shelter; it was a symbol of our resilience, our hope, our survival.

The challenges weren't just physical; they cut deeply into our emotional lives. Every hospital stay, every difficult appointment, every moment we feared for Lion's future brought us to our knees. I remembered the first time I held him after his birth, a moment of profound joy shadowed by the battles we knew lay ahead, yet through the fear, I discovered a strength within me I didn't know existed. I learned I could endure more than I'd ever imagined, that I could be an unyielding advocate for my child and that love could shine, undimmed even in the darkest hours.

During those early days, Milo and Hugo, became unexpected sources of comfort and joy. They navigated the situation with a surprising resilience all their own, anchoring us in ways I hadn't foreseen. Milo, with his nurturing heart, often entertained Lion during those slow, quiet recovery days. He leaned over Lion's crib, sang softly and made funny faces, coaxing laughter and squeals out of his baby brother as though it were the easiest thing in the world.

'Milo,' I whispered one evening, watching him as he sat beside Lion's crib, 'thank you for being such a wonderful big brother.'

He looked at me, his face serious yet gentle. 'Lion's my little brother, Mum. I want him to be happy,' he replied simply.

Hugo found comfort in creating his own worlds, often sprawling out on the living room floor, sketching colourful pictures filled with superheroes and fantastical creatures. His art became a testament to his vibrant imagination, a safe space where he could express his feelings in a way words couldn't. 'Come draw with me, Mum!' he'd call, pulling me down beside him. 'Let's make a city!'

In those moments, we escaped together, leaving behind the oppressive gravity of reality for a while to build a universe of colour and adventure.

Their laughter, their innocence and their joy in the smallest of things acted as a healing balm. They reminded me that, no matter how overwhelming the challenges felt, there was still room for laughter and light. Watching them

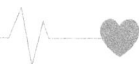

embrace Lion and fill his days with love and laughter, I realised that resilience isn't just about survival; it's about finding reasons to celebrate, even in the hardest moments.

Sitting in the sunlit room, I was filled with gratitude, not only for Lion's progress but for the love and unity that had carried us this far. The journey wasn't over — there would be more hills to climb — but we were ready for whatever came next, bound together by a strength that had carried us thus far. Our home, once a quiet sanctuary, had become a place full of memories, love, and laughter, a place transformed by our journey. I watched Lion play, and as Milo and Hugo joined him, their laughter filled the air, and I knew we'd face whatever lay ahead with strength and togetherness.

The support from family and friends had been my lifeline. Reflecting on those early days, I remembered the endless phone calls, the late-night conversations, and the flood of encouraging messages from all over. My siblings were always there, each call a gentle reminder that I wasn't alone.

'We are here, no matter what,' my sisters, Chloe, Iris and Olive, often said. 'Just pick up the phone if you need anything.'

My friends, Clara and Ava, became my anchors, ensuring I never felt isolated. Clara had an incredible way of calming me with just her voice, lifting me from despair and giving me back a sense of hope. One particularly difficult night, overwhelmed with uncertainty, I received a message from her: 'Just checking in. You're not alone.' That simple text wrapped around me like a warm embrace, giving me strength to face another day. Ava, too, brought her own light into my life. Her unwavering prayers reminded me of the power of faith and friendship. Every caring message, every quick call, was a steady flame that kept the darkness at bay.

Tee, was by my side through it all. Together, we'd navigated the maze of hospital visits, sleepless nights, and the constant strain of not knowing what tomorrow would bring. When I reached my breaking point, Tee would step in to soothe Lion, cradling him close, whispering words of comfort, giving me a moment to catch my breath. 'I've got this,' Tee would say softly, holding Lion with gentle confidence.

Looking back, each challenge transformed me, building a resilience I hadn't known I possessed. I became more compassionate, more attuned to others. Being Lion's mother opened my eyes to the silent battles many families endure. Each time I connected with another parent, sharing

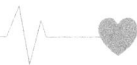

our fears and triumphs, I felt a spark of hope. The bonds formed in moments of shared vulnerability reminded me that we were never truly alone in our struggles.

Our journey taught me to live with gratitude, to cherish the smallest moments: the way Lion's eyes lit up when he saw his favourite toy, the sound of his laughter filling the room, the quiet, peaceful snuggles we shared. Each day felt like a gift, a reminder of life's preciousness. Every evening as I settled into bed, I took a moment to reflect on the day's positives, big or small. That ritual became my way of grounding myself, of choosing to focus on the light.

The sleepless nights in the NICU and PICU taught me patience and perseverance. I vividly remember that sterile environment, the quiet beeps of the machines, the antiseptic smell, the hum of footsteps in the hallway. Those nights were long, each one stretching endlessly, but they strengthened my resolve to fight for Lion's health. I learned to celebrate victories and to find joy amid uncertainty.

Reflecting on one of Lion's extended hospital stays, I remembered Milo and Hugo turning his sterile room into a lively play zone. They had brought blankets, pillows, and toys, transforming the space into a whimsical haven.

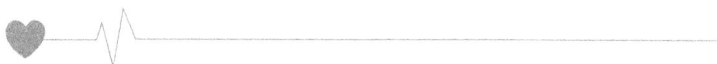

They'd created a makeshift fort and declared it their 'basecamp' for an imaginary adventure, their giggles echoing through the room. Watching them, I was struck by the resilience and pure joy of childhood, and their ability to find magic in the smallest of things.

The journey with Lion also brought me closer to our community. I became involved with local support organisations dedicated to helping families manage complex health issues. At support groups, I met parents who intimately understood the endless challenges of hospital life and medical uncertainties. Hearing others' stories, I felt the responsibility to share my own, to offer hope and support to those who might feel as lost as I once did. Over time, the connections I made turned strangers into friends, each of us contributing to a mosaic of shared resilience.

As Lion grew stronger, I felt profound gratitude for the medical professionals who cared for him. Their compassion, expertise, and dedication were an unwavering foundation, helping us navigates each challenge. One nurse in particular stood out in my memory. She explained everything directly to Lion, making him feel included and safe in a situation that must have been bewildering. Her gentle demeanour brought comfort, and her patience eased our anxieties. I often thought of the doctors and

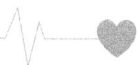

support staff, knowing their commitment to Lion's well-being went beyond just medical care.

As I watched Lion play, his laughter filling our home, I couldn't help but wonder what the future held. The road ahead may have its share of challenges, but I felt ready. I carried with me the strength we'd gained as a family and the love that sustained us through every twist and turn. The sun dipped below the horizon, painting the sky in shades of pink and orange. I took a deep breath and felt a calm wash over me. The journey had been long and often daunting, yet it was filled with love, laughter, and countless blessings. I was grateful for every connection, every hard-earned lesson and every small victory along the way.

I looked over to see Milo reading to Hugo, his voice animated, and my heart swelled with pride. Milo and Hugo had taught me more about perspective than I ever imagined. Their ability to find beauty in the everyday inspired me to embrace life with that same outlook. I remembered one rainy afternoon when we were all stuck indoors, with our moods mirroring the grey skies, then Milo's eyes lit up with an idea. 'Let's build a blanket fort,' he exclaimed, his excitement contagious. Before long, there were pillows and blankets scattered across the living room, transforming our space into a cosy hideaway.

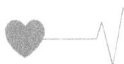

We spent hours in that fort, sharing stories, playing games, and simply enjoying each other's company. That day taught me that even when life felt bleak, we had the power to create our own joy, our own worlds filled with light and laughter.

Even in our hardest times, we wove warmth and love into our days, filling them with moments of joy and connection. Watching my children grow and play, I realised that each giggle, each shared glance, was a precious gift. Life had shown us that while we couldn't always control the road ahead, we could choose how we walked it. Together, as a family, we would keep rising, finding happiness in our own way, and holding tightly to one another through it all. We were a family shaped by resilience and bound by love, and despite everything, I wouldn't trade our path for anything. We would continue navigating life's beautiful chaos, cherishing every miracle along the way.

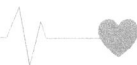

CHAPTER 22

Embracing the Gift of Now

Standing on the threshold of our new chapter, I was enveloped in a sense of optimism that felt both unfamiliar and exhilarating. Looking back, the journey we'd travelled had been fraught with heartache, uncertainty and moments that tested every fibre of my being. There were days when the fear felt insurmountable, when the weight of the unknown loomed large and cast shadows over the simplest of joys, but woven into that tapestry of hardship was a deep, profound joy and a love that I could have only imagined before. Every trial, every victory sculpted us, shaping our family into something stronger and more resilient. As I looked ahead, I was filled with

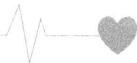

a new hope for the future and an overwhelming gratitude for the present.

Watching Lion grow into his was like witnessing a miracle in slow motion. His spirit was unbreakable; it shone through in every step, every laugh, every moment of curiosity. He became a symbol of resilience, facing each day with a strength that both humbled and inspired me. Seeing him wake up each morning, ready to explore the world with an open heart and boundless energy, filled me with awe. He wasn't just surviving—he was thriving, defying the limitations that once haunted my thoughts. In his growth, I found my own healing. Lion transformed our home into a sanctuary of hope and laughter, and through him, I learnt what it meant to live fully in the moment.

As a family, we discovered depths of strength and compassion I never knew we had. The trials we faced together fortified our bonds, creating connections that went beyond words. Tee and I grew as partners, learning to navigate the complexities of parenthood, stress and uncertainty with newfound empathy and resilience. We leaned on each other, held each other up in our weakest moments and learned to communicate openly, always putting our family's well-being above all else. Our journey deepened our relationship in ways I never anticipated, and I was profoundly grateful for the unwavering support and love we shared. Knowing we could face those challenges together made the future feel less daunting and infinitely more hopeful.

Now, as I prepared to step back into the workforce, I felt a renewed sense of purpose I didn't have before. My journey with Lion ignited a fire within me, a desire to help others facing similar challenges. The support we received along the way was invaluable, and I felt an immense responsibility to pay it forward. I wanted to share our story not only to raise awareness about congenital heart conditions but also to remind others that hope and resilience are possible, even in the face of uncertainty. There is a power in connection, in knowing you're not alone in your struggles, and I wanted to be that source of support for others who were walking similar paths.

I'd already started reaching out to community organisations, exploring ways to get involved and support families dealing with medical challenges. My dream was to create a space—both online and in person—where families could come together, share their stories and lift each other up. Healing, I've come to learn, often began with the sharing of stories and finding understanding in the experiences of others. I envisioned support groups filled with compassion and strength, places where parents

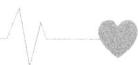

could lean on each other in their darkest moments and celebrate their triumphs, big and small.

In addition to working with families, I committed to creating a strong, supportive community for my own children. Milo and Hugo showed incredible resilience throughout our journey, and we established a tradition of family conversations where we talked openly about our emotions, our dreams, and the challenges we faced. Those conversations became the cornerstone of our family's healing. I encouraged Milo and Hugo to express themselves, to know that their voices were heard and valued. The open dialogue fostered a sense of security and unity, reminding us all that we are navigating on our journey together, bound by love and a shared resilience.

Our outings, once clouded by anxiety, took on new meaning. A simple trip to the park became a cherished adventure, a chance to bond, laugh and savour the beauty of life. Every outing reinforced our belief in the power of joy, in the strength that love and laughter brought to our lives. When I watched Lion play with his siblings, his laughter filling the air and blending with theirs, I was reminded that joy could exist alongside challenges, that love could flourish, even in adversity.

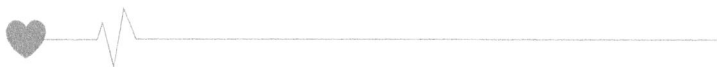

One of my deepest joys was watching Milo and Hugo with Lion. They adapted, evolved and showed strength and compassion beyond their years. Milo, my eldest, took on a gentle, protective role, guiding Lion with patience and understanding. He was a natural nurturer, often helping Lion with tasks or explaining the world to him in ways that surprised me. I saw the pride in Milo's eyes as he taught Lion new things, their bond deepening with every shared moment. Hugo, on the other hand, brought an infectious energy into our home. He had an innate gift for finding joy in the smallest of things, breaking out into silly dances or filling the room with laughter just when we needed it most. Together, Milo and Hugo brought a warmth to Lion's life that was irreplaceable and watching them grow close as brothers filled my heart in ways words could hardly capture.

Our home became a sanctuary of togetherness, and we created traditions that reinforced our bonds. Family game night became one of our most cherished rituals, when we gathered around the table, snacks in hand, and dove into games that brought out our playful sides. Milo was strategic, always thinking several moves ahead, while Hugo's unpredictable choices led to endless surprises and laughter. Lion, still learning the rules, contributed his own unique 'modifications,' and we all laughed until our sides hurt. Those evenings were more than just playing games;

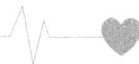

they were a celebration of our resilience, a reminder that even after everything we'd been through, we could still find joy in each other's company.

Cooking together became another beloved tradition. Milo had a knack for experimenting with recipes, Hugo eagerly assisted, and Lion tried to mimic our movements, his little hands grabbing at ingredients with uncontainable enthusiasm. Our kitchen was filled with laughter, with spills and 'uh-ohs,' but those were the moments that made our house a home. They reminded me that love was often found in the simplest acts, in stirring a pot together, in the smell of something delicious baking, in the warmth of shared laughter.

I found myself captivated by the details that once went unnoticed. I saw Lion's eyes light up when he saw his siblings; I heard their laughter blending, a melody that soothed my soul. Each moment was a reminder of the beauty in the ordinary, of the extraordinary strength our family had built. With Lion's health improving, the shadows of worry that once loomed over us were fading, and I was learning to live in the 'what is', embracing today's joys rather than tomorrow's fears.

Stepping into the next chapter, I felt a calling to make a difference beyond our family. I wanted to bring the empathy, resilience and strength I'd found on our journey to my work and every individual I encounter along the way. My experiences with Lion equipped me with more than just professional skills; they gave me an understanding of how vital compassion and connection were in times of crisis. I was ready to be a source of support, to offer hope and guidance to others, knowing firsthand the importance of having someone who understood.

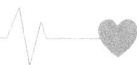

Epilogue

Today, Lion's laughter fills our home, a sound that echoes the resilience and strength he's shown throughout his journey. Every joyful sound, every step, is a testament to the battles he's fought and the miracles we've witnessed together. Watching him thrive, I am overcome with gratitude and awe. His steps are our victories, his smiles our celebrations. He is a living reminder that even the most daunting challenges can give rise to something beautiful. Being his mother is the greatest honour of my life, and I treasure every moment I get to hold him close, feeling the weight of love and triumph in every embrace.

Our journey has transformed us in ways I never could have imagined. It wasn't just about surviving the storm—it was about emerging from it with a newfound strength, compassion, and an unwavering hope that illuminated the

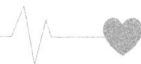

path forward. We didn't just face the hardships; we grew through them, learning to cherish the quiet moments, the small victories, and the deep connections we've forged along the way.

This story isn't just ours. It belongs to everyone who walked beside us: family, friends, medical teams, and even strangers who offered their support when we needed it most. It's a story of hope, love, and resilience—the powerful, unbreakable bonds of family that guided us through the darkest times.

As we step into the future, I do so with a heart full of gratitude and hope. The chapter we've written together is not one of struggle alone but one of triumph, transformation, and unwavering love. We've faced the storm and emerged stronger, closer, and filled with an even deeper appreciation for the beauty in every moment.

Thank you for walking this journey with us, for bearing witness to our story. May it remind you that even in the face of the unknown, love, hope, and resilience will always be enough to carry us through, guiding us back home to what truly matters.

Acknowledgements

To Lion, my brave son:
Thank you for teaching me the true definitions of strength and resilience. Your bravery is the lifeline of this journey and a constant source of inspiration.

To my other children, Milo and Hugo:
Thank you for your remarkable patience, resilience and love during a period when the spotlight was on your baby brother Lion's health. Your understanding, strength and kindness got us through. I am extremely proud of both of you, and I am eternally grateful.

To Tee, my partner:
For being an incredible father and my steadfast companion. Thank you for standing by my side, holding my hand and walking every step of this path with me.

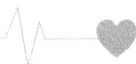

To my extended family, my parents and siblings (my sisters, Chloe, Cora, Olive and Iris, and my brother Finn): Your love, compassion and steadfast support helped me get through every high and low. Thank you for sticking with me and listening to me during my darkest days; I appreciate it.

To my best friends, family friends, and friends: You were my constant support system, offering comfort, strength and a listening ear whenever I needed it. Your presence brought light to the hardest days, and I am endlessly thankful for your kindness and loyalty.

To the healthcare professionals: From doctors and nurses to the dedicated surgeons, physiotherapists, speech and language therapists, play team and care assistants, thank you for your compassion and skill. Your care gave Lion a fighting chance at a healthier life, and I am forever indebted to each of you.

To my university tutors and placement providers: Your understanding, patience and encouragement made it possible for me to continue my education during one of the most challenging periods of my life. Thank you for believing in me.

To Mamita (Tee's mother):
For stepping in with support and care during moments when I felt overwhelmed. Your generosity of spirit brought comfort and strength when I needed it most.

To my employer:
Thank you for your understanding, support and extra time off that allowed me to focus on what mattered most without fear for my job.

My heartfelt gratitude goes out to each of you for playing a part in this journey. I could not have done it alone.

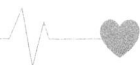

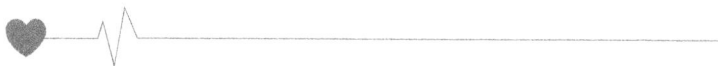

About the Author

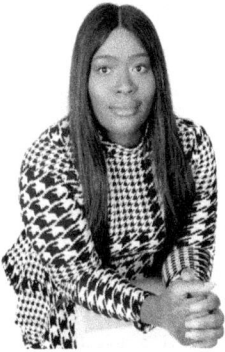

Ezinwanne Lilian Ozuloha is a university graduate, social worker, Wife and mother whose personal journey inspires her heartfelt writing. Her debut memoir captures the profound challenges and triumphs of raising her son Lion, who was born with a cardiac condition. Through this deeply personal narrative, she explores themes of resilience, hope, unconditional love, and the critical importance of support systems.

In addition to her work as a writer, Ezinwanne is the founder of **Radiant Rise**, a social media platform created to inspire hope in others. Drawing from her own experiences, she encourages those facing difficult situations to believe in the light at the end of the tunnel.

Based in the UK, Ezinwanne balances her roles as a writer, social worker, and mother with grace and determination. Her work is a testament to the transformative power of hope, strength, and community.

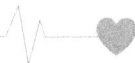

Connect with Ezinwanne:

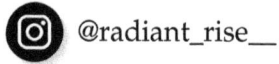

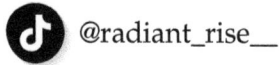

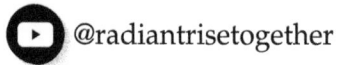

📷 @radiant_rise__

♪ @radiant_rise__

▶ @radiantrisetogether

Conscious Dreams
PUBLISHING

Transforming diverse writers
into successful published authors

www.consciousdreamspublishing.com

authors@consciousdreamspublishing.com

Let's connect

www.ingramcontent.com/pod-product-compliance
Ingram Content Group UK Ltd.
Pitfield, Milton Keynes, MK11 3LW, UK
UKHW050645120525
5863UKWH00046B/744

9 781917 584272